Working in Health and Social Care

For Churchill Livingstone

Commissioning Editor: Susan Young
Development Editor: Catherine Jackson
Project Manager: Derek Robertson/Frances Affleck
Designer: Judith Wright/Keith Kail
Illustrator: Jonathon Haste

Working in Health and Social Care

An Introduction for Allied Health Professionals

Edited by

Teena J. Clouston MBA PGDip(Research) DipCOT DipCouns ILTM

Senior Lecturer, Wales College of Medicine, Biology, Life and Health Sciences, Cardiff University

Lyn Westcott MSc BSc DipCOT RegOT

Senior Lecturer, Wales College of Medicine, Biology, Life and Health Sciences, Cardiff University

Forewords by

Annie Turner TDipCOT MA FCOT

Head of Division of Occupational Therapy, Centre for Health Care and Education, University College, Northampton

and

Nigel Palastanga MA BA FCSP DMS DipTP

Pro Vice Chancellor, Learning and Teaching, Cardiff University

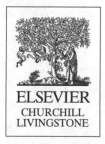

ELSEVIER
CHURCHILL
LIVINGSTONE

EDINBURGH LONDON NEW YORK OXFORD PHILADELPHIA ST LOUIS SYDNEY TORONTO 2005

ELSEVIER
CHURCHILL
LIVINGSTONE

First published 2005

ISBN 0443 074887

British Library Cataloguing in Publication Data
A catalogue record for this book is available from the British Library

Library of Congress Cataloging in Publication Data
A catalog record for this book is available from the Library of Congress

Notice
Knowledge and best practice in this field are constantly changing. As new research and experience broaden our knowledge, changes in practice, treatment and drug therapy may become necessary or appropriate. Readers are advised to check the most current information provided (i) on procedures featured or (ii) by the manufacturer of each product to be administered, to verify the recommended dose or formula, the method and duration of administration, and contraindications. It is the responsibility of the practitioner, relying on their own experience and knowledge of the patient, to make diagnoses, to determine dosages and the best treatment for each individual patient, and to take all appropriate safety precautions. To the fullest extent of the law, neither the Publisher nor the editors assume any liability for any injury and/or damage.

The Publisher

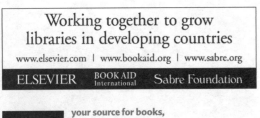

ELSEVIER your source for books, journals and multimedia in the health sciences

www.elsevierhealth.com

The
Publisher's
policy is to use
paper manufactured
from sustainable forests

Printed in the UK

Contents

Part 3: Professional influences on practice

Part 4: First steps into practice

Contributors

Martin Booy MA BA DipCOT TDipCOT ILTM
Dean of Healthcare Studies and Director of Occupational Therapy
Education, Wales College of Medicine, Biology, Life and Health Sciences,
Cardiff University, Cardiff

Teena Clouston MBA PGDip(Research) DipCOT DipCouns ILTM
Senior Lecturer, Wales College of Medicine, Biology, Life and Health Sciences,
Cardiff University, Cardiff

Deb Hearle MSc DipCOT CertEd(HE) DIPISM ILTM
Deputy Director, Occupational Therapy, Wales College of Medicine, Biology,
Life and Health Sciences, Cardiff University, Cardiff

Helen Hortop DipCOT DBA
Honorary Fellow, Cardiff University, Head of Occupational Therapy Services,
Cardiff and Vale Trust, Cardiff

Ritchard Ledgerd BScOT (Hons)
International Manager, Reed Health Group, London

Linda Lovelock BA(Hons) PhD DipCOT
Senior Lecturer, School of Health Professions, University of Brighton

Tracey Polglase MSc DipCOT PGCE(HE) PGDip ILTM
Deputy Programme Manager, Wales College of Medicine, Biology, Life and
Health Sciences, Cardiff University, Cardiff

Gwilym Wyn Roberts MA DipCOT PGDip(Psych) FICP
Deputy Director of Occupational Therapy, Wales College of Medicine, Biology,
Life and Health Sciences, Cardiff University, Cardiff

Robin Sasaru
Clinical Audit Manager, Walsall Teaching Primary Care Trust, Walsall

Soma Sasaru
Clinical Audit Assistant, Walsall Teaching Primary Care Trust, Walsall

Yvette Sheward
Director of Clinical Governance and Training, Walsall Teaching Primary Care
Trust, Walsall

Elizabeth Stallard BA(Hons)Law
Senior Solicitor at Welsh Health Legal Services

Lyn Westcott MSc BSc DipCOT RegOT
Senior Lecturer and Programme Manager, Wales College of Medicine, Biology, Life and Health Sciences, Cardiff University, Cardiff

Steven W. Whitcombe MSc BA(Hons) BSc(Hons)OT PGCE(PCET) ILTM
Lecturer in Occupational Therapy, Wales College of Medicine, Biology, Life and Health Sciences, Cardiff University, Cardiff

Paul K. Wilby MEd BEd(SpEd) MCSP DipTP CertEd(FE)
Director of Interprofessional Education, Wales College of Medicine, Biology, Life and Health Sciences, Cardiff University, Cardiff

Foreword

All allied health professionals who work within health and social care in the UK should be advised to reflect on the words of Johann Wolfgang von Goethe, the 18th century German dramatist, who wisely wrote 'What we do not understand we do not possess.'

The health and social care organisations within the UK are amongst the biggest employers in the world. To practise within them, therefore, is both a unique and common experience. Because of their size, their relationship to central and local government and their place in the national consciousness, health and social care in the UK have developed their own cultures, systems and philosophies, and these impact in a very real way on the day-to-day practice of the people who work in them.

To practise effectively in any situation it is vital to have not only knowledge, but also an understanding of the context in which that practice takes place. To practise in ignorance of the pressures, powers and drivers of the organisation in which you work is to deny both yourself and those who access your service, full use of your knowledge and skills. If we concentrate only on the issues of the people we serve then as practitioners we will be at the whim and behest of the organisation which employs us. To understand both the macro and micro drives and cultures within health and social care, to understand its politics, policies, changes and philosophy, is not only essential for effective practice but also enables us to have some control and influence over that section of the system in which we practise. Therapists who can positively use and influence the context in which they practise are those who will best serve the public for whom they work.

To be an effective practitioner within health and social care requires a knowledge and understanding of how the system sees, and what it requires of its practitioners. The culture that exists within both the organisation and the country has high expectations of its practitioners. Its expectations of autonomous, ethical, effective, evidence-based, professional practice stem from its understanding of professional working. To be effective, therefore, requires practitioners to have a level of understanding and commitment to these principles in order to develop and deliver a service that will best serve the public who own it.

Choosing to enter health and social care within the UK requires not only a commitment to becoming a public servant but also an understanding of how to develop a career pathway that best serves the talents and aspirations of the individual. Practitioners who successfully develop their career are those who will continuously develop and use their talents to the full. Career development within a large organisation offers many and varied opportunities. However it also requires individual professionals to have a knowledge and understanding of the organisation in order to ensure their best pathway through it.

A text such as this, therefore, that helps allied health professionals to understand the context of health and social care in the UK and their unique position within it, will be an invaluable source of reference. To be able to access a text that helps build a clear and dynamic view of the culture and systems in which they are working is one that will help each practitioner towards more effective and efficient practice. As Francis Bacon famously wrote in 1597 'Knowledge itself is power.' To best serve the public from within a large organisation practitioners need to have a clear understanding of their place within it, and this timely text will certainly help the process of making sense of and therefore practising most effectively within the ever-changing health and social care organisations.

Annie Turner TDipCOT MA FCOT
Head of Division of Occupational Therapy
Centre for Health Care and Education
University College, Northampton

Foreword

The title of this book explains very accurately what it contains, and the content must be of interest to a whole range of professional groups. It will be particularly relevant to newly qualified practitioners and final year students who have, or are preparing to, embark on their career in one of the allied health professions. Unfortunately the term allied health professions (AHPs) can hide the fact that there are some strong professional 'tribes' and it is my hope that this book is seen as truly multi-professional as the content is relevant to many, and the profession of the authors is of little relevance.

Teena Clouston and Lyn Westcott have assembled a range of experts who have all made a significant contribution to this text. As editors, Lyn and Teena have managed to keep control of academics and practitioners – which has been likened to herding cats – by introducing and summarising each of the four sections of the book themselves. From my own experience of editing multi-author books, establishing consistency of style without taking away the unique nature of the individual contributions is important. I think the editors have achieved this very difficult task and the end result is commendable.

The book is made up of four sections. Part 1 – *Setting the Scene for Practice* is made up of three chapters covering contexts, systems and change. Part 2 – *Development of the Professions and Individual Practitioner* has four chapters and covers sociological perspectives, teamworking, continuous professional development and development of the allied health professions. Part 3 – *Professional Influences on Practice* has four chapters covering quality, evidence-based practice, audit and legal influences. Part 4 – *First Steps into Practice* has two chapters and appropriately covers preparing and developing your work and securing a post for employment.

From these section headings it can be seen that the authors have managed to cover most areas that surround practice. I think this is the real strength of the book as it appreciates the context within which the reader will operate, but does not get hung up on the intricacies of individual professions. This is not an occupational therapy book written for occupational therapists and should not be seen as such. As a physiotherapist by profession but currently having responsibility for a wide range of medical and socially related professions, I would encourage the reader to consider the content in the way the editors and contributors intended, as a text aimed at helping the health professional. The editors and individual authors should be pleased with what they have produced and I commend this book as a very relevant text for those about to qualify or in the early part of their career. More experienced health professionals might also find it illuminating.

Professor Nigel Palastanga MA BA FCSP DMS DipTP
Pro Vice Chancellor
Learning and Teaching
Cardiff University

Acknowledgements

Our thanks are extended to all the contributors without whom this text would not have been possible.

To all our colleagues whose support over the last year has been invaluable in maintaining the momentum.

To all our students for giving us the ideas and necessary experience.

To Michael, William and George, a patient and supportive family.

To Daniel for encouragement and support.

Dedication

For our friend Claire:
'May your soul and spirit fly'.

Introduction to the contexts of health and social care

Lyn Westcott and Teena J. Clouston

This book has emerged from our experience in the education of allied health professionals (AHPs), particularly student occupational therapists. As tutors we were aware that students, especially as they neared qualification, struggled to find a suitable textbook examining the key areas that contextualised their study of profession-specific skills. Although there were a range of very useful sources examining profession-specific practice, philosophy and theory, there seemed to be little available covering the breadth of subjects needed to help AHPs understand and prepare for practice in the contemporary climate of health and social care. These were issues pertinent beyond our own profession and of common interest to all the professions in the AHP group.

This book has been designed to address this gap drawing on a wide range of areas that need to be understood, in addition to the practice skills that each AHP can offer. Recognising that many readers are likely to be using the book to find out about topics for the first time or wanting to know why the information held in the text is relevant to them, we have designed the structure of the publication so that it can be used in different ways.

The text groups what might be seen as disparate areas into parts, each containing linked themes. An introduction and conclusion are used to help readers think through the relevance of these parts, highlighting how the topics link together and may be applied to the single practitioner, their profession and employing organisation and finally the wider context and setting of British health and social care. Readers may choose to read the book from cover to cover, but are more likely to look at single parts or chapters in a sequence relevant to their needs at the time.

We have encouraged our contributors to enhance their text by ensuring their chapters challenge the reader to be interactive with the material. This has been undertaken in slightly different ways throughout the book, but you will find some interesting illustrative examples across professions, be challenged with reflective questions and posed with exercises that will help bring the text alive and make it relevant to your particular working circumstances.

We hope the book will help readers develop a general understanding of issues across a range of areas and stimulate further interest to examine the topics contained in greater detail and depth. With this in mind, many contributors have recommended further reading or websites that readers can use to develop their knowledge.

It is important to remember that this is an introductory text written about topical issues that are subject to continuous review, development and change.

As such, readers are advised to think through how issues contained here may have been further developed and impacted upon by political drivers, policy changes and professional developments since the date of publication. This should help to ensure that the text retains its relevance and usefulness as a resource to support practice.

PART I Setting the scene for practice

Introduction

Lyn Westcott and Teena J. Clouston

This first part of the book sets out to examine some key areas to help you to understand the wider picture in which an individual practises. These areas are:

- The context of health and social care (Chapter 1).
- Using systems-thinking in health and social care (Chapter 2).
- Working within a process of change (Chapter 3).

To help you organise your thinking and understanding of these complex issues, you may find it helpful to consider how this impacts on your practice from three perspectives.

As an allied health professional (AHP), the most immediate domain of concern for you is usually the individual practitioner and this is important. Understanding your practice, however, is shaped by other, wider domains. The most immediate of these will be the organisation in which you work and the profession to which you belong. These are vital considerations and should be the concern not only of managers but of staff at all levels. Understanding organisational and professional concerns therefore will help you make sense of your practice.

The widest domain considered in this part of the book is that of the whole context of health and social care. By this we mean the political, social and more recently technological factors that influence how health and social care is both shaped and perceived in the UK.

In order to make sense of Part 1, you are advised to bear in mind the three domains outlined above. This will help you understand why the text is relevant to your individual practice. These themes are revisited within the conclusion and summary found at the end of Part 1, which includes an illustration of the key areas within Chapters 1 to 3 under these headings.

1

The context of health and social care

Teena J. Clouston

Not even the apparently enlightened principle of 'the greatest good for the greatest number' can excuse indifference to individual suffering. There is no test for progress other than its impact on the individual. If the policies of statesmen . . . do not have for their object the enlargement and cultivation of the individual life, they do not deserve to be called civilised.

Aneurin Bevan (*cited by Tessa Jowell 1998*)

LEARNING OUTCOMES

This chapter sets out to enable the reader to gain:
- An understanding of the structures of health and social care in the UK.
- An insight into why health and social care changes.
- An understanding of the impact of changes in health and social care on the individual practitioner, the profession and the organisation.

INTRODUCTION

For health and social care, the 21st century has heralded major structural and cultural change. Consequently, understanding the concepts surrounding structure and delivery can be a challenge, not only because of the state of constant flux but because the strategies (or plans) explaining the new ideas are complex and veritably littered with jargonised words. Health and social care is a political animal, not only because it has to meet insatiable demand with finite resources, but because it incorporates and is shaped by political reforms. In other words, the government drives change in health and social care. Indeed, even as political parties write their manifestos so begins another wave of proposed ideas that can instigate another process of evolutionary or even revolutionary change in health and social care arenas.

Although it is this political framework that drives change, it is worth noting that reciprocally, political ideas emerge from environmental, social, economic or technological factors. These elements overlap and work synergically in health and social care to cause movement and change (see Figure 1.1). Consider the following examples:

The World Health Organization (1998) highlighted a need to have a high quality and more integrated health and social care provision. This prompted current thinking in social and therefore political arenas and strengthened the agenda for partnerships, primary focused care and quality in the UK.

Strategies in research and development (Department of Health [DoH] 2001) both harness and create technological advancements (DoH 2003a).

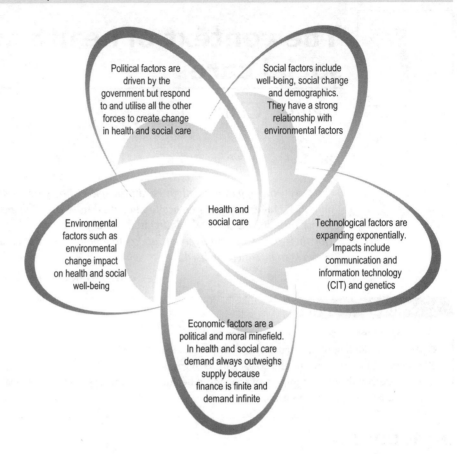

Figure 1.1
Factors impacting on health and social care. Political factors drive change in health and social care but are both shaped by and linked to these other factors.

Social and environmental factors in health promotion have resulted in the government putting more money into health improvement schemes by creating health action zones (DoH 1999).

Demographics, such as the increasing older population, are a direct result of improved health, technological advancement, social and environmental factors. Conversely this has increased the demand on health and social care to meet the needs of older people and maintain their independence (economic factors).

Political reform and developments can both create and enhance services. For example, the modernisation agenda created change and enhanced quality and user involvement. The Freedom of Information Act 2002 and the equalities and diversity document (DoH 2003b) have focused change in certain aspects of services to enhance provision.

The government then, is challenged to balance demands on health and social care with a growing expenditure to meet social needs and a widening, participative agenda. In this way contemporary thought, ideas, developments and available money underpin both what is possible and what is expected from health and social care delivery.

DEVOLUTION

Devolution created an opportunity for Wales, Scotland and Northern Ireland to develop health and social care services specifically to meet local needs. As such, different regions in the UK have the freedom to interpret and respond to external drivers in different ways. National guidance such as the national service frameworks (NSFs) can therefore be applied and used locally to meet need rather than a more 'carte blanche' approach. In theory this should provide a more flexible, high quality service because it targets specific local issues and services. However, because interpretation differs working in different parts of the UK can challenge how we perceive and respond to driving forces. It is worth noting that there is a bias in this chapter towards the English model of health and social care because that provided a pivotal point of reference for the work. As such, consider using this as a springboard to explore your own working practice and environment rather than 'fitting' your setting into the contents of the chapter.

WHAT IS THE MODERNISATION AGENDA?

The most far-reaching changes in the NHS since 1948.

Alan Milburn

The modernisation agenda set out a complex collection of ideas and systems for delivering a health and social care service to meet the needs of people in the 21st century (DoH 1997). These ideas were promulgated through command papers, bills and acts of parliament.

Command papers

Command papers are more commonly known as green or white papers. Green papers tend to be consultation documents or proposals open to public debate, while white papers are actual statements of government policy (The Stationery Office 2003). As such, white papers can create a framework to induce change.

Bills

Bills are primary legislation and set out a proposed law to the government for scrutiny and discussion. In health and social care most bills are public because they deal with matters of general public interest (Northern Ireland Assembly [NIA] 2003).

Acts of parliament

A bill becomes an Act when passed as law by parliament (devolved or central) and has received Royal Assent. As such, an Act is statutory and therefore legally binding.

KEY ISSUES IN THE MODERNISATION AGENDA

The modernisation agenda is both multi-faceted and complex. However, it has approached change in health and social care in the following five key ways:

- Structural change centralised around a primary focused service.
- Integration and joint working through partnerships, not only between health and social care but also voluntary and private sector providers and service users.

- Quality through the models of clinical governance and best value. These promoted a clinically effective, evidence-based service and considered monitoring systems.
- Regulation of the professions to ensure accountability and protection of the public and service user.
- The change agenda for staff. This included radical changes to pay structures, job descriptors, responsibilities and roles.

These common themes are relevant to all aspects of working in health and social care; however, there are fundamental differences in how local interpretation impacts on implementation. As a result the following describes common themes that may apply in subtly different ways in your context.

STRUCTURAL CHANGE

In line with the modernisation agenda, structural change has occurred in all parts of the UK and continues to develop. This dynamic movement is further compounded by devolution as local interpretation and models of service delivery differ. This section attempts to provide an overview of the general concepts underpinning structural change and offer a brief description of local service provision. However, as structures are in a constant state of flux and debate, the aim is to provide a platform for your own research, thinking and application.

Primary care

As a result of the White Paper The New NHS: Modern, Dependable (DoH 1997) and the NHS plan (DoH 2000), (and their Welsh, Scottish and Northern Irish equivalents) local changes in practice and models of working have been focused around a primary care-led service. This has resulted in a service guided by primary care professionals and service users to respond to, and meet local needs preferably in the individual's own home.

Primary care is a term used to encapsulate the first point of contact for service users and thus incorporates general practitioners and other professionals who now provide this service for users. Because of the nature of primary care the interface with social care is vast and integration is unavoidable if high quality service provision is to be achieved. It was this need to work together that, in part, prompted the emerging model of primary care commissioning and management of health and social care provision at local level. These integrated teams represented both primary and social care arenas in a co-ordinated decision-making capacity.

Scotland, Northern Ireland, England and Wales all have slightly different terminology, role definitions and membership of their primary care commissioning teams (Figure 1.2). However, the basic principles driving their inception and priorities were the same – high quality, local, accessible and integrated services (DoH 2000). As a result, primary care focused teams (i.e. teams working as a first point of contact for users) are expanding exponentially. This, consequently, means a change of practice for all allied health professionals (AHPs) either to work in primary care settings or to incorporate that focus and priority within their daily practice in other settings.

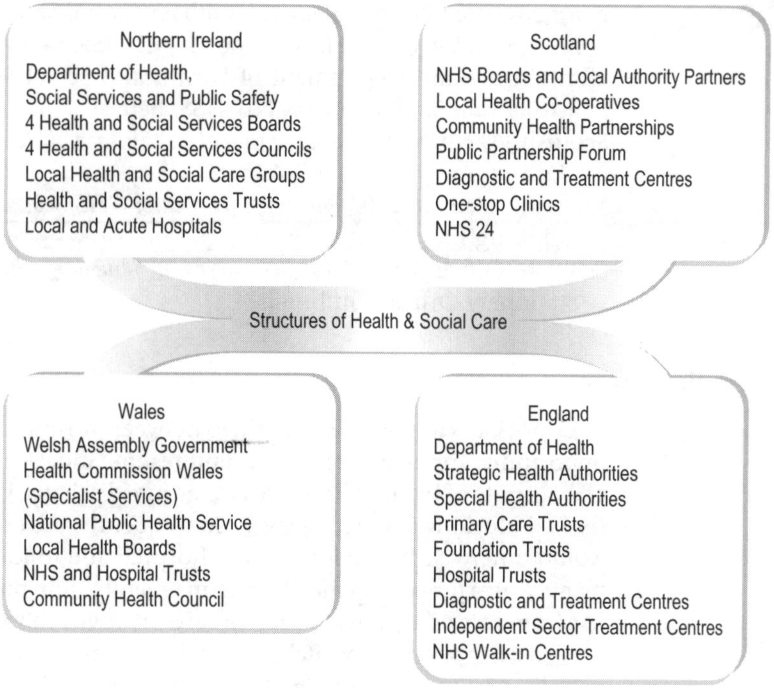

Figure 1.2
Structures in health and social care. These structures are in a constant state of flux – they grow, change and adapt to trends locally, nationally and internationally.

Northern Ireland
Department of Health,
Social Services and Public Safety
4 Health and Social Services Boards
4 Health and Social Services Councils
Local Health and Social Care Groups
Health and Social Services Trusts
Local and Acute Hospitals

Scotland
NHS Boards and Local Authority Partners
Local Health Co-operatives
Community Health Partnerships
Public Partnership Forum
Diagnostic and Treatment Centres
One-stop Clinics
NHS 24

Structures of Health & Social Care

Wales
Welsh Assembly Government
Health Commission Wales
(Specialist Services)
National Public Health Service
Local Health Boards
NHS and Hospital Trusts
Community Health Council

England
Department of Health
Strategic Health Authorities
Special Health Authorities
Primary Care Trusts
Foundation Trusts
Hospital Trusts
Diagnostic and Treatment Centres
Independent Sector Treatment Centres
NHS Walk-in Centres

Social care

Social care is a term used to encapsulate a wide range of support and care services. This includes social services provided by local authorities and care services by voluntary and private agencies. Social care provides services for people who need help to live as independently as possible in the community and people who are vulnerable or need protection. Social care providers work within a framework of duties, responsibilities and national standards set out by central government (DoH 2002).

Key documents

Department of Health 1997 *The new NHS; modern, dependable.* Department of Health, London.

Department of Health 1998 *Modernising social services.* Department of Health, London.

Department of Health 2000 *The NHS plan.* Department of Health, London.

National Assembly for Wales 1998 *Building for the future.* The Stationery Office, Cardiff.

National Assembly for Wales 1998 *Putting patients first.* The Stationery Office, Cardiff.

National Assembly for Wales 2001 *Improving health in Wales: a plan for the NHS with its partners.* The Stationery Office, Cardiff.

Northern Ireland Department of Health and Social Services (NIDHSS) 1999 *Fit for the future: a new approach.* NIDHSS, Belfast.

Northern Ireland Department of Health and Social Services 2000 *Report of the acute hospital review group* (Hayes Report). NIDHSS, Belfast.

Northern Ireland Department of Health and Social Services 2001 *Building the way forward in primary care*. NIDHSS, Belfast.

Scottish Executive 2001 *Our national health: a plan for action, a plan for change*. The Stationery Office, Edinburgh.

Scottish Executive 2003 *Partnership for care: NHS Scotland*. The Stationery Office, Edinburgh.

Scottish Office 1997 *Designed to care: renewing the NHS in Scotland*. The Stationery Office, Edinburgh.

Intermediate care

Intermediate care provides a bridge between hospital and home and offers an opportunity for people to recover and resume independent living more quickly. The purpose of intermediate care is to ensure discharge home safely while preventing bed blocking at hospital level. Consequently, the emphasis is on people who would otherwise have a long stay in hospital and follows comprehensive assessments with a timed, specific, short-term rehabilitation programme and as such, differs from secondary care. Models of service provision vary. It may, for example, be provided in a specific hospital or unit where intensive rehabilitation is needed after a stroke, or it may take the form of a rapid response, re-ablement or a hospital-at-home team. Intermediate care works on an integrated basis with primary care teams, social care staff and hospital-based services to ensure that people have active support to enable independence at home. In this way intermediate care teams can also be utilised for assessment and intervention with a view to preventing a potential hospital admission. Intermediate teams can be composed of staff from a variety of employers and settings and work across traditional boundaries.

Key documents

Department of Health 2001 *Intermediate care HSC2001/01:LAC*. Department of Health, London.

Department of Health 2001 *The national service framework for older people*. Department of Health, London.

Community services

Community services are usually associated with NHS trusts and are community-based teams working in partnership with social services. For example, this may include community mental health teams, learning disability teams or physical disability community teams. Local areas differ in their definitions of what constitutes community care in the light of the primary care initiatives.

Secondary care

This is specialist care usually provided by a hospital. This can include acute or community type hospital services. Intermediate care teams often support discharge from hospital and thus work in tandem with secondary care services.

Tertiary care

Tertiary care encapsulates specialist units or hospitals providing care for specific or complex conditions or illnesses requiring long-term support.

Hospital trusts/NHS trusts

Hospital and NHS trusts provide a range of care services and interventions in a variety of settings. They offer specialist services or have areas of expertise utilised regionally or nationally. Community services are often managed by trusts.

NHS direct

This is a 24-hour, nurse-led helpline providing confidential advice and information on symptoms, health concerns, self-help and support organisations. The national number is 0845 4647.

NHS online

This is the online link to a mine of information:

http://www.nhsdirect.nhs.uk/	(England)
http://www.nhsdirect.wales.nhs.uk/	(Wales)
http://www.show.scot.nhs.uk/	(Scotland)
http://www.n-i.nhs.uk/	(Northern Ireland)

Because the structures in each devolved area of the UK differ, it necessary for you, as a practitioner, to associate yourself with the structure best suited to your needs (see Figure 1.2). Ideas around structure and delivery continue to develop in line with clinically effective, evidence-based strategies and are therefore dynamic. Your professional body, organisation, newspapers, journals and relevant web sites will enable you to keep up to date. The local models offered below can only offer a provisional guide for your own research and understanding.

THE ENGLISH MODEL

In the English model, the primary care-based commissioners of health and social care are called primary care trusts (PCTs). These teams or boards of people comprise general practitioners, primary care staff, service users and health and social care representatives. Their remit is to make collaborative decisions about the focus of health and social care in the local area.

Care trusts

Care trusts were first announced in the NHS Plan (DoH 2000). They represent a joint venture in health and social care provision and deliver integrated, whole systems (see Chapter 2 for systems theory) services as a single organisation. The legal framework for care trusts was set out in Section 45 of the Health and Social Care Act 2001, and built on existing partnership working afforded by the Health Act 1999 flexibility arrangements. Care trusts have a single management structure and multi-disciplinary teams managed from one point, a shared location for staff, and a single, cross-disciplinary assessment process. In most instances budgets are pooled and services are arranged around joint equipment stores. As such, service configuration is integrated and ensures a streamlined service from hospital to home. Although there is flexibility to determine service provision at a local level, care trusts tend to focus on specialist mental health and older people's services.

Foundation trusts

Foundation trusts have caused controversy amongst health and social care employees and unions because of concerns about independence in decision making and the possible consequence of creating a two-tier system in competition with NHS trusts. This perceived threat is linked to the three fundamental differences foundation trusts have from other trusts. These are:

- They are legally independent entities separate from the Department of Health. As a result, foundation trusts can make decisions about spending money. However, they are still subject to review by an independent regulator.
- They have the power to raise finances from independent sources.
- Local people are active members of the board of governors.
- The Health and Social Care (Community Health and Standards) Bill (2003) advocated the inception and provided the authority for foundation trusts.

Diagnostic and treatment centres (DTCs)

DTCs were first mentioned in the NHS Plan 2000. They were designed to address waiting lists and provide alternative avenues for elective surgery and diagnoses.

Because the specific nature of the work is elective and routine, DTCs can supposedly provide constant levels of work, unaffected by the seasonal variations that occur in NHS hospitals due to increased emergency admissions.

Independent sector treatment centres (ISTCs)

These were planned as an independent service and designed to address waiting lists and to offer an alternative to DTCs. Service users therefore have greater choice in accessing services. Although managed by private companies, these services remain free of charge to NHS users.

NHS walk-in centres

NHS walk-in centres provide an easily accessible, 7-day-a-week service for everyone. They provide advice, basic treatment and intervention, assessment by nursing staff, advice on healthy living, information on out-of-hours GP and dental services and information on how to access allied health professions.

Strategic health authorities (SHAs)

Strategic health authorities manage the NHS locally and are a key link between the Department of Health and the NHS. They oversee the functions of PCTs and trusts, are responsible for developing strategies for local health services and ensuring high-quality performance. They also ensure that national priorities (such as the NSFs) are addressed.

Special health authorities

Special health authorities have a similar role to SHAs but oversee health services to the whole population of England not just a local community, e.g. the National Blood Authority.

THE WELSH MODEL

The Welsh Assembly Government (WAG) oversees the provision of health and social care in Wales. The structure and associated terminology differs from the English model but both share the common factor of ongoing change. NHS trusts work closely with local authorities and other partners to provide stream-lined, primary focused health and social care services. Both trusts and local authorities have a remit to support local health boards with the development of a health, social care and well-being strategy for Wales.

Local health boards (LHBs)

LHBs are the health and social care commissioning teams in Wales. The LHBs and their corresponding local authorities have a duty to work together and in partnership with other local agencies to provide high quality, local and accessible services. This includes the development of intermediate and community service provision. LHBs also have a remit to develop a joint health, social care and well-being strategy for Wales.

The national public health service (NPHS)

The NPHS is a single organisation that provides advice and guidance for the LHBs on public health and well-being.

Community health councils

This organisation assures service user involvement at all levels of service provision.

Health Commission Wales

The Health Commission Wales is responsible for providing advice and guidance to LHBs on acute hospital, specialist or regional services, for example cancer services.

Key document

National Assembly for Wales 2002 *Improving health in Wales: a plan for the NHS and its partners*. The new NHS Wales functions and structures.
Online. Available:
http://www.wales.gov.uk/healthplanonline/health_plan/index.htm#scp
28 November 03.

THE SCOTTISH MODEL

The White Paper Partnership for Care (Scottish Executive 2003) and the NHS Reform Scotland Act 2004 proposed radical changes to health and social care provision in Scotland. This included abolition of NHS trusts and a unified NHS board and the development of a special health board called Health Scotland to consider health and well-being in this region.

NHS boards

NHS boards work with local authority partners to develop partnership agreements to provide integrated, local community, primary focused service provision. These services work with specialist healthcare providers through clinical and care networks. These networks can cross professional boundaries and provide an integrated, single pathway of care for service users. Scotland in particular, utilises managed care networks (MCNs) to organise integrated systems of care for users.

Community health partnerships (CHPs)

LHCCs represent a diverse group of people and develop into community health partnerships. These services have the responsibility to plan and develop devolved local services in Scotland and form effective partnerships with the local authority services. They form a focal point for integration and have greater influence over the deployment of resources by NHS boards. Reciprocally, NHS boards have a monitoring role over both local health co-operatives and community health partnerships.

Scottish Health Council

The Scottish Health Council monitors the performance and effectiveness of the health boards.

The Scottish Executive

The Scottish Executive further enhances and assures quality service provision in Scotland.

Diagnostic treatment centres

DTCs have a similar role to those in the English model and offer a wider range of services to Scotland.

One-stop clinics

One-stop clinics represent an integrated community and primary care service and a partnership between NHS boards, local authorities and other partnership organisations such as the police or voluntary agencies.

Local public partnership forums

These public/user-led organisations assure user presence in the local community health partnerships.

Key document

NHS Reform Scotland Act 2004.
Scottish Executive 2003 *Partnership for care*. NHS Scotland. The Stationery Office, Edinburgh.

THE NORTHERN IRELAND MODEL

The model of health and social care in Northern Ireland has a more integrated approach known as health and personal social services. Health and social services trusts (HSS trusts) are the providers of health and social services. They manage staff and services at ground level and control their own budgets. However, as in other areas of the UK, this model is open to change.

Health and social services boards (HSSBs)

There are currently four HSSBs (Eastern, Northern, Southern and Western) in Northern Ireland. These are responsible for assessing the needs of their respective populations and commissioning services to meet those needs. They are charged with the establishment of key objectives to meet the health and social needs of their population and the development of policies and priorities to meet those objectives.

Local health and social care groups (LHSCGs)

LHSCGs are committees of health and social care boards and link providers of primary and community services. Members include primary care professionals, service users and representatives from health and social services boards or trusts. One member must be an allied health representative.

Health and social services councils (HSSCs)

The four HSSCs monitor health and personal social services. As independent consumer organisations, these councils have a duty to represent the public's views and interests, to review the work of health and social services and to recommend any improvements needed.

Department of Health, Social Service and Public Safety (DHSSPS)

The DHSSPS has a polity role similar to the Department of Health in England. It aims to improve the health and social well-being of the people of Northern Ireland. The four health and social services boards are agents of the DHSSPS in planning, commissioning and purchasing services for the residents in their areas.

THE PARTNERSHIP AGENDA

Bring down the Berlin wall between health and social care.

Frank Dobson

The partnership agenda endorsed inter-agency, inter-professional and service user partnership, a system of working together to provide the best possible care for those accessing services (Scottish Office 1997, DoH 2000). The boundaries of inter-agency working have been pushed to include the private as well as statutory and voluntary sectors. This integrated approach to care has resulted in initiatives such as care pathways and managed clinical networks.

Managed clinical networks (MCNs)

Managed clinical networks can be defined as 'groups of health professionals and organisations from primary care, secondary and tertiary care working in a co-ordinated manner, unconstrained by existing professional and health board boundaries to ensure equitable provision of high-quality clinically effective services' (Scottish Office 1999). As such, clinical networks enhance not only multi-professional working practice but inter-organisational ones. However, MCNs also have a remit to involve service users and carers, set and demonstrate evidence-based standards of service, and ensure that appropriate management is available to sort out difficulties arising in the care of individuals and the networks as a whole. Finally, the network must link to organisational strategy and report the network performance to the public to inform users and maintain a transparency in service provision.

Integrated care pathways (ICPs)

Integrated care pathways are 'both a tool and a concept that embed guidelines, protocols and locally agreed, evidence-based, patient-centred, best practice, into everyday use for the individual patient' (National Electronic Library for Health [NeLH] 2003). The NeLH also states that 'an ICP aims to have . . . the right people, doing the right things, in the right order at the right time, in the right place, with the right outcome all with attention to the patient experience to compare planned care with care actually given.'

As a tool then, care pathways can provide clear guidance to intervention, assure best practice, equitable and integrated provision to service users. Pathways are common practice in the UK and have been developed to encapsulate integrated intervention for specific conditions with service user involvement.

Service user involvement

The involvement of service users in the partnership agenda aimed to promote inclusion and empowerment in decision making. This has impacted on AHPs in several ways. In the first instance, the methods used to keep service users informed have become more transparent. As such, copies of clinical letters written by one professional to another about a service user should be copied to the service user concerned (DoH 2000). Second, the practicalities of the single assessment exercise and the use of pluralistic evaluation tools should, in general terms, enable communication, clarity and understanding for both users and professionals.

Key documents

Community Care and Health (Scotland) Act 2002. HMSO, London.

Department of Health 2000 *Meeting the challenge: a strategy for allied health professionals.* Department of Health, London.
Online. Available:
http://www.doh.gov.uk/iwl/meetingthechallenge.html
27 Oct 2003.

Department of Health 2001 *Intermediate care HSC2001/01: LAC.* Department of Health, London.

Department of Health 2001 *Shifting the balance of power: securing delivery.* Department of Health, London.

Health and Social Care Act 2001. HMSO, London.

Health Act 1999. HMSO, London.

Joint Future Group 2000 *Community care: a joint future.* Scottish Executive.
Online. Available:
http://www.scotland.gov.uk/library3/social/ccjf.pdf
29 Oct 2003.

Scottish Executive 2003 *Partnership for care.* Scotland's Health White Paper. The Stationery Office, Edinburgh.

QUALITY AGENDA

Treat people as if they were what they ought to be and you will help them to become what they are capable of being.

> Goethe

The quality agenda is a cross boundary theme and exists in all services that provide health and social care. Quality was highlighted politically because of issues raised by inquiries into certain incidents in health and social care, for example the Bristol inquiry (Kennedy Report 2001) and the Climbié Report 2003. The English White Paper, A first class service quality in the new NHS (DoH 1998a) introduced the clinical governance model as a means of defining and measuring quality. The Health Act 1999 carried this into statute and as such, all healthcare providers have a duty to provide quality services. In a similar vein the English White Paper Modernising social services (DoH 1998b), introduced the concept of best value as a quality measure for local authorities (and therefore social care) and the Local Government Act 1999 made this statute. Both concepts share similar themes and are monitored by external bodies. Under the Health and Social Care (community health standards) Bill 2003, the new Commission for Health Audit and Inspection (CHAI), to be known as the Healthcare Commission, was given responsibility for healthcare while the Commission for Social Care Inspection (CSCI) monitors social care. Although differences in implementation and terminology exist at local level, the drive for quality is universal and includes concepts such as clinical effectiveness, evidence-based practice, risk management, professional leadership and service user involvement and participation as high priority elements.

National service frameworks (NSFs)

National service frameworks provide guidance on the implementation of key priorities for health and social care services and their partners. NSFs provide national standards, service models and guidance in the implementation of best practice. They also provide a framework against which performance can be measured. There are several NSFs, all highlighting priority areas for health and social care delivery. These include mental health, older people, children's services, coronary heart disease, diabetes services (standards and delivery), the national cancer plan, renal services and long-term conditions. Although the standards in the NSFs are national there are some differences in interpretation in devolved parts of the UK to accommodate demographics and local need.

Key documents

Department of Health 1999 *Clinical governance – quality in the new NHS*. Department of Health, London.

Department of Health 2000 *A quality strategy for social care*. Department of Health, London.

Department of Health 2000 *Meeting the challenge: a strategy for allied health professionals*. Department of Health, London.
Online. Available:
http://www.doh.gov.uk/iwl/meetingthechallenge.html
27 Oct 2003.

Department of Health 2002 *National service frameworks – a practical aid to implementation in primary care*. Department of Health, London.

NHS Information Authority 2003 *NSF information strategies – NHS information authority*.
Online. Available:
http://www.nhsia.nhs.uk/nsf/pages/default.asp
26 Nov 2003.

Welsh Assembly Government 2002 *National service frameworks in Wales*.
Online. Available:
http://www.wales.nhs.uk/sites/home.cfm?orgid=334
26 Nov 2003.

THE AGENDA FOR CHANGE (AfC)

As a term, the agenda for change has become synonymous with changing roles and pay structures for staff in health and social care.

Pay structures

The pay structure is a single eight-band pay scale with salaries ranging across a wide differential. Individual staff are linked to the appropriate band through matching their job description to the job profiles in the AfC structure. These profiles are based on 16 measures, categorised by job knowledge and skills, role responsibilities and requirement for physical and mental effort.

Changes in roles

As health and social care services adapt to meet need, so working practice needs to change accordingly. Models of service provision, extended practice, flexibility, training and development, lifelong learning, clinical specialist and consultant therapist posts are just some of the ways in which these changes are emerging. The government has highlighted 10 key roles as a framework for AHPs to enable change in practice as follows:

- To be a first point of contact for patient care, including single assessment.
- To diagnose, request and assess diagnostic tests and prescribe, working with protocols where appropriate.
- To discharge and/or refer patients to other services, working with protocols where appropriate.
- To train and develop, teach and mentor, educate and inform AHP and other health and care professionals, students, patients and carers, including the provision of consultancy support to other roles and services in respect of patient independence and functioning.
- To develop extended clinical and practitioner roles which cross professional and organisational boundaries.
- To manage and lead teams, projects, services and case loads, providing clinical leadership.
- To develop and apply the best available research evidence and evaluative thinking in all areas of practice.
- To play a central role in the promotion of health and well-being.
- To take an active role in strategic planning and policy development for local organisations and services.
- To extend and improve collaboration with other professions and services, including shared working practices and tools.

These roles represent a key strategy to implementing change in AHP working practice and highlight a need for clinical specialism, clinical leadership, involvement in policy development and expansion in roles and responsibilities. Prescribing is not as contentious at it first appears as all AHPs already have the ability to provide medication under a patient-specific direction (PSD), i.e. a written instruction from a doctor or dentist. Some AHPs (chiropodists, orthoptists, physiotherapists, radiographers, ambulance paramedics and optometrists) can also provide medication under patient group directions (PGDs), a written instruction for the supply or administration of medicines to a group of patients rather than an identified individual (DoH 2003c).

Regulation of the professions

The NHS Plan 2000 introduced the concept of health regulators to regulate individual health professions as part of the government's plan for modernising the NHS. This was supported by the findings of the Bristol Royal Infirmary Inquiry (The Kennedy Report) 2001. Contemporaneous to this the Health Act 1999 introduced powers to reform and modernise the existing systems. The National Health Service Reform and Healthcare Professions Act 2002 set out the functions of the Health Professions Council (HPC) for the regulation of health-care professionals and its powers and duties. These include providing a framework that enables:

- Putting patients' interests first.
- Being open and transparent to allow public scrutiny.
- Being responsive to change.
- Provision of greater integration and co-ordination between the regulatory bodies and the sharing of good practice and information.
- Regulatory bodies to conform to principles of good regulation.
- Regulatory bodies to act in a more consistent manner.

These changes impact on AHPs in several ways but the following describes two of the key issues raised through regulation.

Protection of title

Since July 2003, professionals registered with the HPC have had 'protected' titles. This means that non-registered individuals cannot call themselves an art therapist, music therapist, drama therapist, art psychotherapist; medical laboratory technician (biomedical scientist); chiropodist, podiatrist; clinical scientist; dietician; occupational therapist; orthoptist; prosthetist, orthotist; paramedic; physiotherapist, physical therapist; radiographer, diagnostic radiographer, therapeutic radiographer; speech and language therapist or speech therapist. This both protects the validity of the profession and professional, and more importantly assures protection for service users. It is likely that this list will expand over time as even more professions join the HPC registers.

Accountability

The NHS Plan 2000 proposed that accountability to the public and the professions was the key to effective reform of regulation. As a result regulatory bodies such as the Health Professions Council, have to ascertain and demonstrate that they are acting in the public's interest and prioritising the protection of service users. Moreover, they have to actively enable public involvement at policy and procedure level and balance this with meeting the needs of healthcare providers. For individual practitioners this means we are both protected and responsible for protecting the rights and interests of service users.

Key documents

Department of Health 2001 *Modernising regulation in the health professions consultation document.*
Online. Available:
www.doh.gov.uk/modernisingregulation
18 Nov 03.
Department of Health 2002 *Human resource performance framework.* Department of Health, London.

CONCLUSION

The government agenda impacts on both professional and organisational structure, strategies (including aims and outcomes), culture, systems, policies and procedures. It therefore has an effect on both professional practice and organisational agendas. As such it impacts on professional bodies and health and social care organisations by providing a framework for how they think, plan and move forward in developing their services for the future. This, in turn, impacts on individual practitioners by shaping how they work, reason, achieve expected outcomes and develop professional roles and behaviours.

Working in different areas around the UK can modify the impact or emphasis of the agenda. As such it can be a challenge for professionals to maintain an overview across the whole country. As individual practitioners, you need to be aware of the nuances in your own area of work and the differences that might occur if you move into a different part of the UK. Finally, however, the health and social care environment is dynamic and constantly changing; to keep up to date is an ongoing task but one necessary to maintain the expectations of a professional working in health and social care in the 21st century.

Reflective questions:

■ *Why does the UK government drive change in health and social care?*
■ *How do the changes in health and social care impact on your profession?*
■ *What do these changes mean for you as an individual practitioner?*
■ *What are the key issues that impact on practice as a result of professional regulation?*
■ *How has the structure of health and social care changed from that described in this chapter?*

WHERE TO FIND INFORMATION

The internet is a key facility as this is updated regularly. Also your professional body and employing organisation can provide you with updated information and frameworks.

Useful websites

Bulletin for Allied Health Professions
http://www.doh.gov.uk/ahpbulletin/

Department of Health
http://www.doh.gov.uk or http://www.doh.gov.uk/index.htm

Gateway to Health and Social Care (Northern Ireland)
http://www.n-i.nhs.uk/

Health Professions Council
http://www.hpc-uk.org

Health and Social Care Joint Unit
http://www.doh.gov.uk/jointunit/

Health of Wales Information Service
http://www.wales.nhs.uk/

HMSO
http://www.hmso.gov.uk/

Integrated Care Network
http://www.integratedcarenetwork.gov.uk/

Mental Health Act Commission
http://www.mhac.trent.nhs.uk/

Modernisation Agency
http://www.modern.nhs.uk/scripts/default.asp?site_id=10

National Institute of Clinical Excellence
www.nice.org.uk

Northern Ireland Government
http://www.ni-assembly.gov.uk/

National Health Service
http://www.nhs.uk/

Public Health Electronic Library (Phel)
http://www.phel.gov.uk/index.html

Scottish Parliament
http://www.scottish.parliament.uk/

Scottish Executive Health Department
http://www.show.scot.nhs.uk/

The Stationery Office
http://www.official-documents.co.uk/menu/command.htm

UK Parliament
http://www.parliament.uk/

Welsh Assembly Government
http://www.wales.gov.uk

REFERENCES

Department of Health 1997 *The new NHS: modern and dependable*. Department of Health, London.
Department of Health 1998a *A first class service: quality in the new NHS*. Department of Health, London.
Department of Health 1998b *Modernising social services*. Department of Health, London.
Department of Health 1999 *Saving lives: our healthier nation*. Department of Health, London.
Department of Health 2000 *NHS Plan: a plan for investment, a plan for reform*. Department of Health, London.
Department of Health 2001 *Research governance framework for health and social care*. Department of Health, London.

Department of Health 2002 *Frequently asked questions about social services*.
Online. Available:
http://www.doh.gov.uk/cos/frequentquestions.htm
27 Nov 2003.

Department of Health 2003a *Our inheritance, our future – realising the potential of genetics in the NHS*. Department of Health, London.
Online. Available:
www.doh.gov.uk/genetics/whitepaper.htm
02 Oct 2003.

Department of Health 2003b *Equalities and diversity: strategy and delivery plan to support the NHS*. Department of Health, London.
Online. Available:
http://www.doh.gov.uk/nhsequality/strategydocumentoct031003.pdf

Department of Health 2003c *Supply and potential future prescribing of medicines by allied health professionals*. Department of Health, London.
Online. Available:
http://www.doh.gov.uk/chpo/prescribing.htm
Nov 28 2003.

Freedom of Information Act 2002 HMSO, London.

Health Act 1999 HMSO, London.

Health and Social Care Act 2001 HMSO, London.

Health and Social Care (community health and standards) Bill 2003 HMSO, London.

Jowell T 1998 *Nye Bevan Memorial Lecture – a third way for public health*. Published: Monday 29th June, Reference number: 98/264.
Online. Available:
http://www.dh.gov.uk/PublicationsAndStatistics/PressReleases/PressReleasesNotices/fs/en?CONTENT_ID = 4024652&chk = IU47aV.
23 Dec 2003.

Local Government Act 1999 HMSO, London.

National Health Service Reform and Healthcare Professions Act 2002. HMSO, London.

National Electronic Library for Health (NeLH) 2003. *About integrated care pathways*.
Online. Available:
http://www.nelh.nhs.uk/carepathways/icp_about.asp#what
28 Nov 2003.

Northern Ireland Assembly 2003 Assembly Legislation
Online. Available:
http://www.ni-assembly.gov.uk/legislation/legislation2000.htm
30 Oct 2003.

Scottish Office 1997 *Designed to care: renewing the NHS in Scotland*. The Stationery Office, Edinburgh.

Scottish Office 1999 *The introduction of managed clinical networks within the NHS in Scotland*. Management Executive Letter Circular MEL. The Scottish Office Department of Health, Scotland.

Scottish Executive 2003 *Partnership for care: NHS Scotland*. The Stationery Office, Edinburgh.

The Report of the Bristol Royal Infirmary Inquiry 1984–1995 (The Kennedy Report) 2001. Cmnd Paper 5207.
Online. Available:
http://www.bristol-inquiry.org.uk/index.htm
18 Nov 2003

The Stationery Office 2003 Command Papers
Online. Available:
http://www.official-documents.co.uk/menu/command.htm
18 Nov 2003.

The Victoria Climbé Inquiry 2003 HMSO, Norwich

World Health Organization 1998 *Health for all in the 21st century*.
Online. Available:
http://www.who.int/archives/hfa/index.html
27 Oct 2003.

RECOMMENDED READING

Allsop J, Saks M 2002 *Regulating the health professions*. Sage, London.
* An in depth academic book looking at the legal, ethical and professional implications of regulation for health professions and professionals.
Dawes M et al. 1999 *Evidence-based practice. A primer for healthcare professionals*. Churchill Livingstone, Edinburgh.
* A good overview of evidence-based practice and its implications for practitioners in healthcare.
Hill A (ed) 2000 *What's gone wrong with health care? Challenges for the new millennium*. Kings Fund, London.
* A basic text looking at some of the dilemmas in decision making and service provision for the NHS. It utilises a case study approach and considers the human aspect of care.
Lugon M, Secker-Walker J 2000 *Clinical governance. Making it happen*. Royal Society of Medicine, London.
* A practical guide to clinical governance and its implications for practice. It highlights best practice in implementation and considers diverse issues such as integrated care, clinical audit, risk management and complaints. Also contains a useful guide to other sources.
Ovretveit J 2002 *Evaluating health in interventions*. Open University Press, Buckingham.
* A really useful and contemporary introduction to evaluation in health care, considering a variety of methods and approaches.
Swage T 2000 *Clinical governance in healthcare practice*. Butterworth Heinemann, Oxford.
* A good introductory text to clinical governance and the wider quality agenda.

JOURNALS

As well as your professional journals:
Therapy Weekly is a key read for any allied health professional.
The Health Service Journal is a weekly magazine full of interesting information, articles and facts for health managers and staff.

Using systems-thinking in health and social care practice

Martin J. Booy

INTRODUCTION

Systems science and systems-thinking, with origins in biology, engineering management science, has produced various methodologies to assist in understanding complexity and inform complex problem solving. In the context of health and social care, a basic appreciation of systems-thinking and concepts can help understanding of, for example, the way professional models of practice are designed. Organisations can be described in systems terms. Some working practices and procedures seem to work well whilst others can be dysfunctional. A systems approach can be used to design coherent policies and procedures and also to check the robustness of existing practices in a logical way.

SO WHAT IS A SYSTEM?

A system can be described as an assembly of components linked together in an organised way. The components are affected by being in the system and the behaviour of the system is changed if they leave it and this assembly of components has been identified as being of particular interest. Finally, this organised assembly 'does something' and some 'emergent property' is evident as a result.

For example, consider a common brick (Figure 2.1). (Yes, a brick, a piece of fired clay measuring about 23 cm long, 10 cm wide and 7.5 cm high with two or three holes in the middle.) What could you use it for?

The obvious response would be 'for building a wall', but others might suggest' 'a pen holder, a flower pot, a wheel chock'. The more bizarre might even think of a brick as a teething aid (as in the context of 'chewing a brick'), as an aid for burglary or as a weapon. However, in all these examples, the brick is nothing on its own. Each of us will make a judgement based on our own knowledge to place this brick in context. Thus a car driver might visualise the brick as a wheel chock,

Figure 2.1
A common brick.

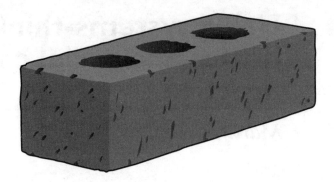

because it may help solve a problem of parking a car on a hill; the potential burglar may see it as ideal to smash the window of the local jeweller's shop. The view that a brick is used for building may have less relevance to an inhabitant of the equatorial jungle than those who live within a community where brick built homes are common.

However, when considering the various options for using a brick, all will involve the brick as a component part of something greater. For example, for a brick to operate successfully as a wheel chock, the other components such as a wheel (of a vehicle), a force acting on the wheel (such as gravity) and the brick need to be linked together in an organised way to make the 'system' work effectively. Placing the brick wheel chock on the downhill side of the wheel will enable the system to achieve its 'purpose' of preventing the wheel rolling down the hill, rather than if you placed it on the uphill side of the wheel. Finally, as the owner of a car with a non-functional parking brake, this system may be of particular interest as a temporary solution until a repair can be effected. (In systems-thinking this known as an emergent property.)

Exercise 1

Try and identify the components and purpose of the other 'systems' which could include a brick.

So relationships between the components are important. The order or sequence in which components appear in a system affects the way it works. Historical sayings such as 'shutting the stable door after the horse has bolted' or 'putting the cart before the horse' exemplify the importance that 'doing things in the right order' has had in society. Computers tend to work more quickly, but still depend on processing tasks in sequence albeit at a speed that exceeds human reasoning. The components in these 'systems' are therefore linked together systematically (Checkland 1981) (see Figure 2.2).

Systematic thinking and action are important in the way we carry out our daily activities. Walking, eating, dressing or 'making a cup of tea' are skills we learn as we grow up which involve such sequencing. As health and social care professionals we support individuals in the acquisition or reacquisition of these skills which have been impaired by illness, injury or delayed development. In using a developmental approach to intervention, sequencing or 'chaining together' the stages of a task can be manipulated to promote learning. Systematic action is also important when using technical equipment as a healthcare practitioner.

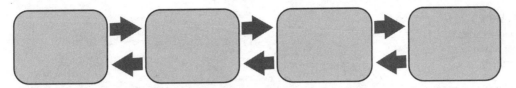

Figure 2.2 Components linked systematically.

Figure 2.3
A professional
practice system.

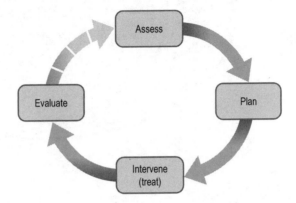

Examples could include the application of radiotherapy or ultrasound. To perform the procedure non-sequentially could prove hazardous to service user and practitioner.

When considering a set of human activity components sequentially, it can be portrayed as a cycle. In describing the stages in a 'professional practice system' as a systematic cycle, the opportunity to reiterate the process in the light of evaluation is given (see Figure 2.3).

However, the sequential or systematic attribute is only one of those needed to place a system in context. Each system will itself be part of a wider system and may also possess sub-systems. Thus they are arranged as a hierarchy, with the smaller systems being sub-systems for the next level up. When considering a system in this way you are analysing it systemically (Checkland 1981) (see Figure 2.4).

Figure 2.4
A systemic
hierarchy of
systems.

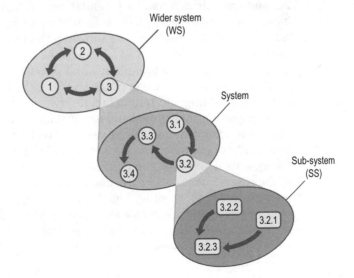

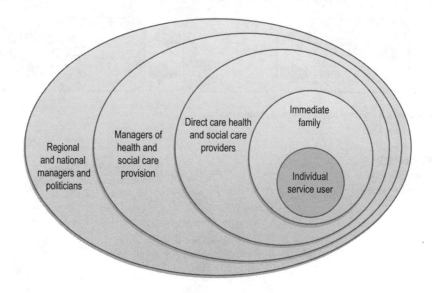

Figure 2.5
An alternative appreciation of hierarchy.

Thus it is possible to view a system in different levels of complexity whilst also portraying the systemic relationships between components at each level of detail. Hierarchical, systemic thinking helps us to understand organisations such as the National Health Service (NHS) in the UK, and to analyse the activity of an individual. However, hierarchy need not just be viewed 'from the top down' as is traditional when building organisational charts. In this case the top layer of the NHS would be the incumbent politician heading the Department of Health or its regional equivalent. This approach places the patient, client or service user at the bottom layer. A more 'person-centred' approach to systemic, hierarchical thinking can place the service user at the centre of the organisation, with the health or social care professionals and family members and carers in the closest supportive relationship (see Figure 2.5).

Therefore, systems-thinking involves the concurrent consideration of systematic and systemic aspects of a potential system. It also helps to structure complexity and to place strategic 'high level' thinking in context with the detail of a sub-system. Within the hierarchy shown in Figure 2.5, the detailed needs of the individual service user are most relevant at the centre of this hierarchical arrangement, involving service user, family and direct care workers. The further away from this central core the less emphasis is given to the individual. The priorities change to enabling and resourcing of service provision with greater emphasis on policy making at regional and national level. Problems arise in the relationships of systems working at these various levels when a component is taken out of context. For example, if a national or local politician (who has contributed to the legislation and policy making at a wider system level) becomes embroiled in the specific issues of a particular service user, they may criticise the implementation of services within 'rules' which they have been responsible for creating! For health and social care managers caught in the middle of such a fracas, such systemic thinking and rationale may be a useful tool to explain their role within the context of a total service provision.

It is also useful to consider the relation between the *what* and *how* in a systems hierarchy. Referring to system S in Figure 2.4, the sub-systems (SS) will give extra detail on *how* the system works. Conversely, the wider system (WS) can clarify *what* the key task of system S is.

SYSTEMS BOUNDARIES

The concept of a boundary is readily used in daily life. Such boundaries may be:

- *Physical boundaries:* The boundary fence around a property, the county boundary, the 'bricks and mortar' of a building.
- *Organisational boundaries:* The boundary which separates membership and non-membership of an organisation. For example, registration of a healthcare practitioner forms an organisational boundary between registrants and non-registrants. However, criteria for membership of the organisation such as employment status or specific qualification, determine the roles and responsibilities of its members.
- *Systems boundaries:* A systems boundary can be either or both of the above, and more. It encloses the 'series of components linked together in an organised way' and helps to clarify the relationship of a particular system with other systems, both systemically and sequentially. Thus, within a 'rehabilitation system', there will be sub-systems which exclusively describe occupational therapy, physiotherapy, nursing (ward) and medical activities within the context of rehabilitation. Systems boundaries will be determined by professional roles and responsibilities, but can also be used to clarify the scope of decision making and control of those who operate the system (Bulow 1989) (see Figure 2.6).

Figure 2.6
System boundaries based on decision-making responsibilities.

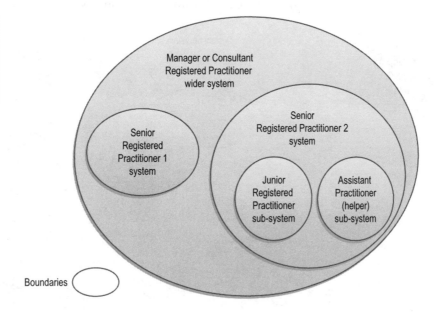

Table 2.1

Decision to be made	Level of decision taking required
1 Professional assessment of patient/client needs	e.g. Junior registered practitioner
2 Identification of care protocol to be used by patients/clients with similar problems or diagnosis	
3 Allocate funds to purchase equipment for service	
4 Decide in which order to see patients when assisting with dressing practice	
5 Allocate junior staff to individual patients/clients	

Overlapping systems boundaries

The use of systems-thinking can be particularly helpful when trying to unravel the complexity of overlapping systems. An example of this can be found at the interface between the health and social care systems within the UK. In Figure 2.7, the components of the process of discharging a service user from hospital into the community are shown as two overlapping systems, S1 and S2. However, there are problems in the relationship between these systems because components X1 and X2 are duplicated and components Y1 and Y2 have been excluded or ignored by the existing systems. X1 and X2 could be the duplication of the same assessment by a hospital professional in S1 and an equivalent professional employed by the local council. Components Y1 and Y2 could be service needs

Figure 2.7 Overlapping boundaries of systems.

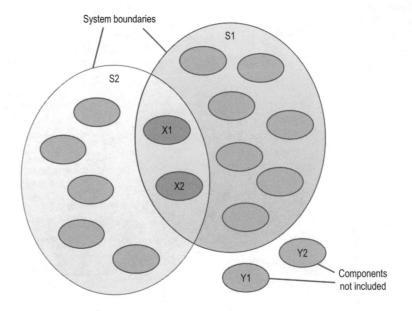

identified for the user being discharged which neither professional sees as their responsibility. Such boundary diagrams can inform negotiation over the recon-figuration of the systems boundaries of S1 and S2 to promote efficiency of effort and inclusiveness of service (see Figure 2.7).

However, overlapping boundaries can be used constructively as well. In Figure 2.8, the service user is placed at the centre of the inter-professional healthcare team. Each professional has a proportion of exclusive uniprofes-sional activities. Some activities can intentionally be carried out by a number of professionals (for example, helping a service user to use the toilet) in the interests of a seamless service and for a more efficient use of staff time. Some activities, such as adhering to a code of professional conduct, will be relevant to all team members (see Figure 2.8).

Monitoring and control

Being a decision-taker within a system implies that decisions taken have influ-ence or control over the system. But to justify changing the behaviour of a system, the functioning of the system needs to be monitored before any control action is taken. In turn, in order to be able to make decisions about changing the behav-iour of the system as decision-taker, clarity is required over the purpose of the sys-tem. (Remember that in first introducing the attributes of a system, one was that the system 'did' something.) In practice, these expectations can include profes-sional benchmarks for performance, care standards, financial performance, or aims and objectives for intervention with a patient/client or user (see Figure 2.9).

Figure 2.8
The overlapping boundaries of the inter-professional healthcare team.

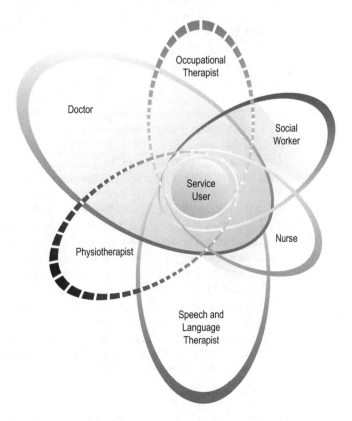

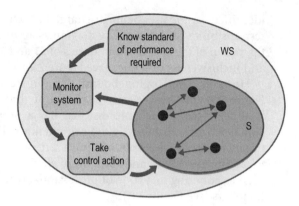

Figure 2.9
The monitoring and control loop of the wider system.

A case scenario

Do we do what we think we do?

To illustrate the various systems principles introduced in this chapter so far, an example is offered from the author's personal experience when carrying out an action research with a colleague as part of a postgraduate study (Booy, unpublished dissertation, 1987). The general manager of a large district general hospital (this would now be called an acute hospital trust) had approached the University for advice regarding a problem with management of the nursing services. The project took place at a time when health professionals were beginning a general management role within the NHS in order to provide a more integrated service. Action research involves working with those directly involved in the situation to help them resolve the uncertainty. Thus the researchers interviewed a wide cross-section of the nursing workforce at all levels from the chief nurse to staff nurses and also met with the hospital administrators and other health professionals.

From this a model of a 'system to manage patient care' was devised as a series of actions (not unlike the professional practice system in Figure 2.3). The main system had about seven components, but when the detail of each component was described at a sub-system level, about 67 sub-component activities were identified. This model was then discussed in a series of focus groups representing different levels within the nursing hierarchy at the hospital, to check that (i) they were in agreement with the model and (ii) which aspects of the model their own job involved. Thus, the nurses (the 'actors' in the system, Table 2.3 refers) agreed by consensus both what they thought *should* happen and their understanding of what *did* happen in reality. This study highlighted that the roles and activities of the ward managers (ward sister/charge nurse) were replicated by their immediate superiors (the nursing officers) in the equivalent of the assessment, planning and implementation stages of the 'patient care management system' but that neither grade was completing the cycle by taking responsibility for the monitoring and evaluation of the effectiveness of this 'patient care management system'.

In systems terms this was portrayed as a significant overlap of systems boundaries, with the evaluation components ignored by both. It also demonstrated confusion

continued

Input →	'Transformation'	→ Output
Patients requiring care	Provide care	Patients provided with care
Care providers needing employment	Employ care providers	Care providers employed
Resources available for care provision	Provide resources	Used resources

Table 2.2

between activities taking place and different levels in the systems hierarchy. The role of the ward manager would be to work with system S in Figure 2.9 and the nursing officer should be operating within the wider system (WS), monitoring the performance of a number of ward manager operated 'systems' within their control.

In the feedback to the management and nursing staff at the end of the project, the overlaying of transparency slides of the ward manager and nursing officer 'systems' on top of a diagram of the 67 agreed activities of their new system to manage patient care, was a graphic illustration to all concerned. It led to reconfiguration of the nursing officer grade job descriptions and justified some management training for the new post holders.

Such a technique could be useful for establishing roles within an interdisciplinary health or social care team (for example a community mental health team), where the intended functions of the team are described in systems terms and then the activities in each member's role would be compared with the team system to identify role overlap and elements which no one performed (see Table 2.2).

SOME RULES FOR BUILDING SYSTEMS

For a system to work effectively, its design will need careful consideration. This mental processing is called conceptual modelling (Checkland 1981), and may result in a number of different interpretations of the potential system. If designing the NHS for the first time, the conceptual models of the NHS from the perspective of a potential service user, a health professional practitioner and the government minister responsible would vary considerably. Therefore a number of models would need to be created, interpreting the 'world view' of each of these stakeholders. If the eventual system needed to be used by all three stakeholders, then some negotiation would be necessary to lead to a consensus agreement.

One advantage of using diagrams to describe a situation is that all elements can be appreciated at once and kept in mind when examining aspects of a sub-system or the wider system. When initially trying to portray an area of interest in diagrammatic form, 'anything goes' and the result can be a 'rich picture' of the unstructured problem (for example see Figure 2.10).

In any systems diagram, relationships of the components (the contents of the bubbles in the diagram) are portrayed by lines and arrows to show the connectivity or communication of the system. It is vitally important to know the nature of this relationship (i.e. what the arrows mean). A simple rule is to be consistent in the way components are identified. They can be either entities (names) or activity statements (which have to include a verb). Thus the words hospital, day centre

Figure 2.10
Building entity
and activity
systems models.

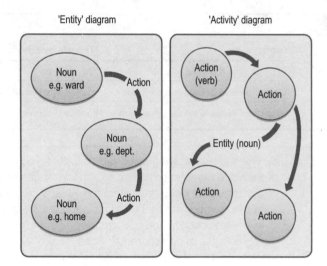

and home could be the named components and the arrows would indicate the movement or actions between them. In an activity diagram, describing a similar relationship, terms such as 'discharge from hospital', 'attend day centre', 'live at home', would comprise the components with facts rather than actions being represented by the arrows (see Figure 2.10).

The problem arises when a diagram does not follow these 'rules'. In following the arrows connecting the components the nature of the relationship between them becomes unclear.

Exercise 3

Build a systems model of your current place of work, firstly as an entity diagram and then as an activity diagram (e.g. how your department is organised).

'What happens in the bubble?' The concept of transformation

The next stage is to consider the detail of the 'relationship' between the bubbles and the arrows. The arrows pointing into a 'bubble' are the *inputs* into the system and the arrows pointing away from (perhaps towards another activity) are referred to as the *outputs*. Therefore the 'activity' that occurs within the 'system bubble' changes an input into an output. This is called transformation, because it changes or transforms an input into an output (Checkland and Scholes 1990) (see Figure 2.11).

For example, if the human activity system is to 'provide patient care', then there will be a number of paired inputs/outputs that contribute to the system (Table 2.2 refers).

Figure 2.11
The
transformation
process.

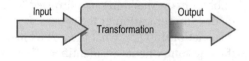

Open and closed systems

A system can be described as either open or closed, depending on whether, once started, it influences and responds to the 'environment' outside the system boundary. A simple example of a closed system would be a set of traffic lights that change every 3 minutes, regardless of the amount and presence of vehicles waiting to move in each direction. This can be changed to an open system by including a movement sensor as a component which will ensure the system responds to changes in the environment. The Model of Human Occupation (Kielhofner 1997) describes individual people as open systems who both influence and adapt to the wider environment. However, in the management of the Health and Social Care Service within the UK it is important that this concept of systems openness is ensured. There is a public perception that NHS and local authority policies and procedures are rigidly observed by health and social care professionals to the detriment of potential users of the service and with no consideration of what is going on outside 'the system'.

METHODOLOGY FOR ACTION

The second part of this chapter introduces a systems methodology that is particularly appropriate for use within the health and social care sector. As with any model of practice, it can be used to frame a problem-solving process through a series of inter-related steps. Remember that systems-thinking is concerned with understanding the complexity of 'whole' situations and this is as important to the novice practitioner as to the strategic manager. Although the original methodology was first designed by Professor Peter Checkland and colleagues at Lancaster University, UK in the 1970s (Checkland 1975, 1981) it is still used in various forms to assist problem solving in settings where the situation is 'soft and messy', that is where the problems are complex and undefined or where you think there is something wrong with a particular system, but you are not sure what. Soft systems methodology (SSM) is a system to structure problem situations and offer possible solutions based on conceptual modelling. In its original, simplest form (Mode 1) it has seven steps to work through (Checkland 1975) (Figure 2.12 refers). However, progress thorough the stages is rarely straightforward and there is usually the need to revisit earlier stages for clarification of detail (known as iteration).

Step 1: The problem unstructured

As a health or social care professional, the first stage of any contact with a service user is to assess the problem situation (this is similar to the first stage of the assessment, planning, intervention, evaluation process). Information is obtained from as many sources as possible: the service user, relatives, other professionals and so on. You may wish to interview various potential stakeholders to obtain their particular view of the problem in order to understand aspects of the problem that are important to them (for example, ensuring the views of service users are included along with those of health professionals if you think there may be a problem with the delivery of a particular service).

Figure 2.12
Soft systems
methodology
(Mode 1)
(Checkland
1975).

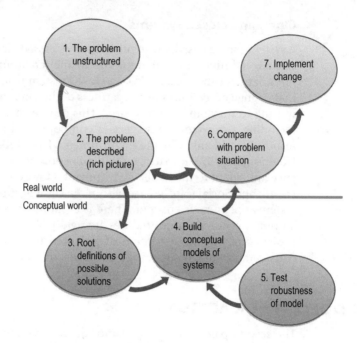

Step 2: The problem described

Having gathered as much information as possible, the problem situation needs to be described holistically (all at once) so that issues and potential conflicts are identified and the relationships between the various actors or processes in the scenario are pictured as a 'rich moving pageant of relationships' (Checkland and Scholes 1990, p. 45). There is no correct way of drawing a rich picture. Some may choose to use a series of words and arrows in the form of a mind map. Others may choose to introduce simple pictorial representations or cartoon 'pin men' to increase the impact. However, the purpose at this stage is to describe the problem holistically, not to begin to build a new system. Have patience in this and observe the rigour of the methodology.

The rich picture in Figure 2.13 attempts to portray the various issues and influences on the members of a local authority social services department who are trying to encourage independent living by their service users, but only seem to make them more dependent on 'the system'. It indicates relationships between those who work for social services, their professional colleagues in the hospital, the service users and their families, the influences of the local community and the effect of government policy and legislation. Although this scenario is based in social services, the issues described are relevant to the wider health and social care sector. The 'system' is not working as intended and everyone is unhappy about it. Users' relatives are complaining to the press and to local politicians because they consider that their nearest and dearest are not receiving the level of service which was expected.

The constraints on the level of service provision to individuals is allocated through a maze of criteria and priorities which seem unfair to service users in need and seen by the staff as placing them in an unfavourable light with their clients. Overlooking the whole scenario is potentially conflicting legislation

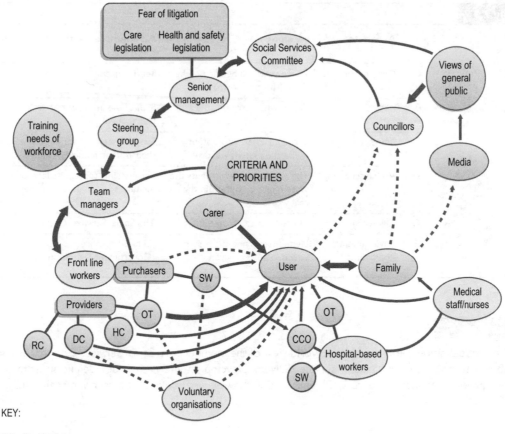

KEY:

RC = Residential care
DC = Day care
HC = Home care
OT = Occupational therapist
SW = Social worker
CCO = Community care organiser

Figure 2.13 A rich picture of a Social Services Department which was seeking to identify the pressures on its staff that influenced effective working practice. After Booy and Boniface (1999).

which, whilst protecting employers within the workplace, contradicts encouraging service users to become more independent (Figure 2.13).

The rich picture also seeks to reflect the particular perspective or world views (weltanschauungen) as they may be held by the various stakeholders. Any new system(s) would need to accommodate the variety of values and beliefs held.

Step 3: Developing root definitions

The purpose of stages 1 and 2 of SSM is to clarify the 'real world' problem scenario. In stage 3 the opportunity is provided to develop root definitions of possible systems to address it. These definitions normally start with 'A system to . . .'

Table 2.3

	Attribute	Meaning	An example for the scenario in Figure 2.13
C	Customer(s)	Those who will be affected by the T (the transformation)	Service users
A	Actors	Those who carry out the T	Staff of the Social Services Department
T	Transformation	Changing input into output (what the system will do)	Support service users in maximising their potential quality of life
W	Weltanschauung	The world view which puts the system into a context in the real world	Society aims to help its less fortunate members
O	Owner(s)	Those who can stop the T	The Social Services Committee
E	Environmental constraints	Elements outside the system which it takes as given	Limited resources Government legislation

Exercise 4

The root definition below reflects the world view of the members of a Social Services Committee and the values that they hold around service delivery. Develop an alternative root definition from the information contained in Figure 2.13, representing the *weltanschauung* of the user and their family.

and include six key elements to ensure the rigour of the statement. Checkland (1981) suggested the mnemonic CATWOE as a check for these (see Table 2.3).

As such, the statements generated by CATWOE can be incorporated into a rigorous definition of a potential system, providing an appropriate level of detail from which to begin to 'build conceptual models' of a potential system. Therefore in working through the given example, *one* root definition could be:

A Social Services Committee owned system which enables its staff to support service users in maximising their potential quality of life, reflecting societal values within the constraints imposed by legislation and resources available.

Step 4: Building conceptual models

Time spent in developing a cogent root definition will then make the next stage relatively simple, ensuring a consistent level of detail appropriate to the place of a system within its systemic hierarchy of wider systems and sub-systems. In a detailed analysis, sub-systems would explain *how* each activity within the system would be achieved (see Figure 2.14).

The example of a conceptual model (Figure 2.14) is intentionally set at a relatively simple level of complexity and could be at the level for decision making by the Social Services Committee. Each of the activities within the model can themselves be developed in more detail as sub-systems. For clarity each component

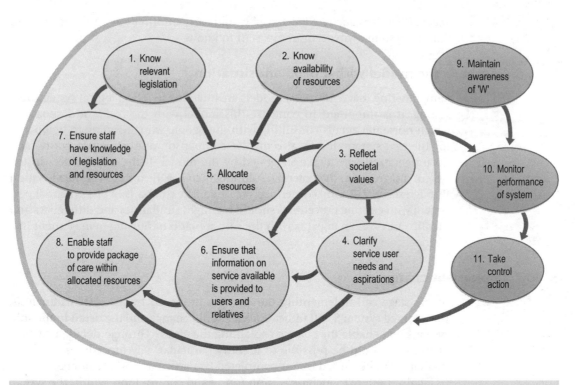

Figure 2.14   A conceptual model of the system described in the sample root definition.

Table 2.4		
Effectiveness	Is this transformation (T) meeting the longer term aim? *(To support users in achieving their potential)*	
Efficiency	The amount of output divided by the resources used *(Costs per staff/user involvement, or cases completed by staff within resources available)*	
Efficacy	Does the system 'do' what is required of it?	

activity should numbered so that any sub-systems of that component can be cross-referenced in the form of a systems hierarchy (Figure 2.4 will remind you of this).

Step 5: Testing the robustness of the model

Before comparing the conceptual model of a possible solution to the problem with the real life situation, it is sensible to check the robustness of the systems reasoning against three criteria, often referred to as the 3 Es: Effectiveness, Efficiency and Efficacy (Forbes and Checkland 1987) (Table 2.4).

Be clear also about what is passing along the 'arrows' between the activities. For example the arrow between *'Know relevant legislation'* and *'Ensure staff have knowledge of legislation and resources*' would carry information on the legislation that the system owner requires its staff to know.

Step 6: Compare the model with a problem situation

Remembering that conceptual models are intended to reflect logical systems reasoning, it is important to compare this model with the real world situation, which normally entails consulting with the people who are going to be operating the new system. It may also involve comparison of existing procedures and documentation with those suggested by the model. If the stakeholders in the system disagree with the potential solution, then it is the time to conduct iteration through stages 2–5 until consensus is reached. The comparison of a potential new system with existing procedures should highlight similarities and differences and identify areas for change (as with the case scenario of nursing management in a district general hospital).

Step 7: Implement change

At the stage of implementing the changes proposed by the systems analysis, the adopted system S will indicate *what* should change and the detail in the subsystems will enable the change explaining the *'hows'*. Through detailed systems analysis, it would be possible to identify particular new procedures, or documentation to be carried out or completed by particular staff members.

Finally, be sure to include a 'monitoring and control loop' within the system design so that the '3 Es' can be regularly checked and the system can maintain its integrity.

CONCLUSION

This chapter has sought to provide an introduction to the world of systems-thinking and its potential relevance to professional practice within health and social care (Chapman 2001). In the first part of the chapter, the elements required to build a system have been described and advice about building systems diagrams and models has been included. The second part of the chapter introduced one systems methodology (Checkland's SSM) in its original Mode 1 form to illustrate how systems-thinking can inform the problem-solving process used by health and social care practitioners.

There is a wealth of information available for those who wish to delve further into systems-thinking. New generations of systems methodologies are constantly being developed; for example, Total Systems Intervention – TSI (Flood 1995). SSM itself has undergone considerable refinement over time (Checkland and Scholes 1990, Checkland and Holwell 1998). The concept of systems-thinking is fully incorporated into information management and technology. Even the National Health Service considers the way forward to be through a 'whole systems approach' (DoH 2000). If you want to develop your skills in systems-thinking, a good place to start is through the courses and publications of the Open University which has been involved in teaching systems for over 30 years. Much of the course work is related to scenarios in the health and social care sector so you may find this both useful and familiar.

REFERENCES

Booy M, Boniface G 1999 Enabling older people. Developing a social-services owned system. In: Castell et al. (eds). *Synergy matters: working with systems in the 21st century.* Kluwer Academic/Plenum Publishers, New York pp. 301–306.

Bulow I von 1989 The bounding of a problem situation and the concept of systems boundary in soft systems methodology. *Journal of Applied Systems Analysis* 16: 35–41.

Chapman J 2001 An introduction to 'systems'. *Systemist – Journal of UK Systems Society* 23: 80–83.

Checkland PB 1975 The development of systems-thinking by systems practice – a methodology from an action research programme. In: Trappl R, Hannika F de P (eds). *Progress in cybernetics and systems research, Volume II.* Hemisphere Publications, Washington.

Checkland PB 1981 *Systems-thinking, systems practice.* Wiley, Chichester.

Checkland P, Scholes J 1990 *Soft systems methodology in action.* Wiley, Chichester.

Checkland P, Holwell S 1998 *Information, systems and information systems.* Wiley, Chichester.

Department of Health 2000 *Working in partnership – developing a whole systems approach.* Project Report. HMSO, London.

Flood RL 1995 *Solving problem solving. A potent force for effective management.* Wiley, Chichester.

Forbes P, Checkland PB 1987 *Monitoring and control in systems models.* Internal discussion paper 3/87. Department of information systems and management. University of Lancaster, Lancaster.

Kielhofner G 1997 *A model of human occupation – theory and application*, 3rd edn. Lippincott Williams and Wilkins, Baltimore.

RECOMMENDED READING

McDermot I, O'Connor J 1997 *The art of systems-thinking.* Harper Collins, New York.
* This introductory reading is recommended by the Open University.

3 | Working within a process of change

Deb Hearle and Tracey Polglase

LEARNING OUTCOMES

This chapter sets out to enable the reader to gain:
■ An understanding of the change process and its impact on the individual and organisation.
■ The ability to understand and utilise a variety of tools to help implement or cope with the change.
■ The skills to effectively evaluate the process and outcome of change.

INTRODUCTION

Whether you are working in the health service, social care, education or the private sector, change will be inevitable. As Hamer and Collinson (1999, p. 182) state 'Whichever organisational culture or structure you work in, the one constant will be change.' Enormous changes have occurred within the working environments of the allied health professions and it appears that this is not isolated to the UK. Terry and Callan (1997) cited in Lloyd and King (2002, p. 536) identified this as an international issue when they state: 'Over the last two decades, Healthcare organisations in the western developed nations have experienced unparalleled change to their structures, procedures and personnel.'

This is further supported by Shervington (2003), who argues that change cannot be stopped and that the challenge for individuals and organisations is not dealing with it, but rather managing the higher and higher levels of change.

You may be a person instigating change, a member of a working group addressing one aspect or you may need to manage or respond to change. Whatever the case is, if change affects you in some way, either directly or indirectly, you will wish to have some influence over its implementation and to do this will need to understand how policies are developed and implemented (Cameron and Masterson 1998). There are many ways of being proactive and embracing changes, and a dynamic professional would always rather be a change-agent than the resistant dinosaur.

This chapter will help you to understand the process of change, how it impacts on the organisation where you practise and what these changes mean to you as an individual practitioner. It will also provide a toolbox of skills to help you to instigate, manage or cope with change. By the end it is hoped that strategies can be adopted which will enable you to view change positively. You should also have an understanding of the many ways in which you can develop ownership of those policies and procedures within your work.

UNDERSTANDING CHANGE

Although much is written on change and its management, there are very few clear definitions. Change can be defined as a continual process of evolution or revolution from one position/perspective to another; the many different contexts make it a very complex issue. The key message to realise is that change is a constant process, and one in which people need to work rather than fight against in order to survive.

Change is essential within an organisation because adaptation is required to:

- Accommodate the changing needs of the service users.
- Meet increasing demands of the organisation.
- Respond to needs identified by research and evidence-based practice.
- Increase effectiveness/efficiency (although this is sometimes difficult to see).
- Cope with imposed changes (e.g. reduction in staffing, legislation).
- Stay competitive within the market.

A number of influences drive change. Lloyd et al. (2002, p. 163) state: 'Internationally there have been major changes in the delivery of healthcare services, influenced by economic, social and political factors.' With this in mind, it is therefore very important that professionals are aware of the chief factors that affect their organisation. To keep up to date with these it may be necessary to incorporate relevant investigative/research activities as part of all therapists' continuing professional development.

In order to categorise the driving forces a PEST (sometimes known as STEP) analysis can been used. PEST is mnemonic for:

- *Political:* Political issues, e.g. legislation, dynamics.
- *Economic:* Macro- and micro-economic trends including issues specifically relating to the purse holders.
- *Social:* Social factors that will affect the service/s, e.g. changing attitudes, demographic changes.
- *Technological:* Advances which may be of benefit.

These broad categories are not discrete and often impact upon one another. Within health and social care the influences could include things such as the increasing older population and legislation. Further examples are illustrated in Figure 3.1.

Figure 3.1
Examples of influences using a PEST analysis.

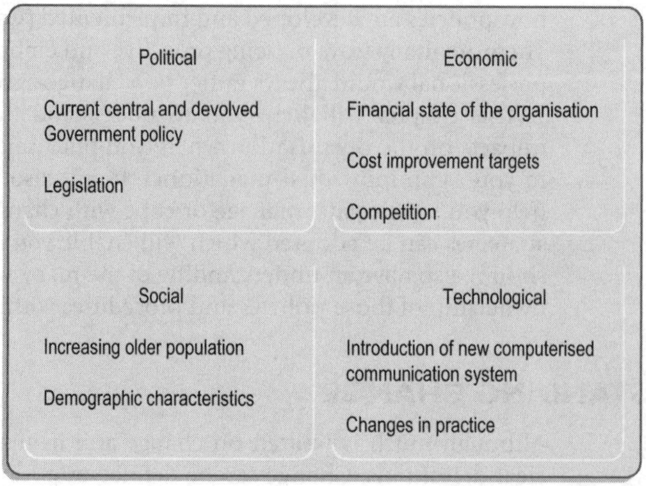

Political	Economic
Current central and devolved Government policy	Financial state of the organisation
	Cost improvement targets
Legislation	Competition
Social	**Technological**
Increasing older population	Introduction of new computerised communication system
Demographic characteristics	Changes in practice

To work within an environment of change, it is important to appreciate the theories and their application. Just like professional models of practice, they help us to clarify and analyse the problems in order to provide a clear route for intervention. This is particularly important for junior practitioners who may require some direction in order to help facilitate or accommodate the process of change.

Hamer and Collinson (1999) identified three basic elements of all models of change:

- Recognition of the need to change (situational analysis).
- Implementation of an action plan for change.
- Period of consolidation and evaluation.

In the following section several models have been outlined which will help you understand change. These are presented under two distinct categories: those that help to explain the change process, and those that highlight the impact upon the individual/organisation.

UNDERSTANDING THE PROCESS

Kurt Lewin (1958) identified two models of change, namely *Force Field Analysis* and the *Unfreezing–Changing–Re-freezing* model. Both describe a similar process involving analysis then problem-solving in that order.

Force field analysis model

Lewin suggests that organisations or situations are held in balance or equilibrium between two sets of forces (see Figure 3.2).

- *Driving forces:* those instigating the change.
- *Restraining forces:* those preventing developments or making them difficult.

Figure 3.2 Application of force field analysis model – starting point.

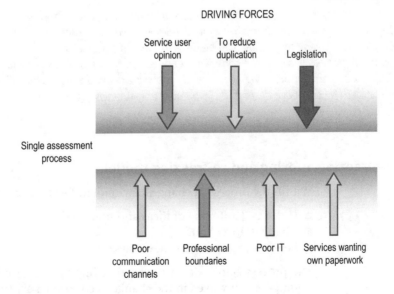

DRIVING FORCES

Service user opinion   To reduce duplication   Legislation

Single assessment process

Poor communication channels   Professional boundaries   Poor IT   Services wanting own paperwork

RESTRAINING FORCES

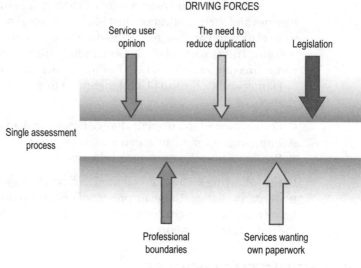

Figure 3.3
Application of
force field
analysis model –
end point.

DRIVING FORCES

Service user opinion

The need to reduce duplication

Legislation

Single assessment process

Professional boundaries

Services wanting own paperwork

RESTRAINING FORCES

When using a force field analysis the impact of the two sets of forces is analysed. In order to achieve change the driving forces must outweigh those that are restraining. The most effective way of achieving this is not to increase the number of drivers but to reduce/manage the restraining forces. Figures 3.2 and 3.3 illustrate this with an example of the single assessment process (see Example 3.1). It is important to note that the aspects identified as driving or restraining forces may have different levels of importance and these are represented in the figures by the size of the arrows.

Example 3.1

The single assessment process is driven by legislation and the need to improve the quality of care for the individual. The resistance to it revolves around individual services wanting their own paperwork and professionals requiring their aspects to be done to their professional standards. If managers were to fully support the process this could be considered to be an additional driving force. However, this would not reduce the concerns of the workforce, whereas improving communication channels and information technology (IT) would have decreased the number of restraining forces and allowed the change to progress more smoothly.

The unfreezing, moving and re-freezing model

Within the process of change, Lewin identifies three crucial phases:

- Unfreeze (softening of ideas and practices).
- Change/movement.
- Refreeze (accepting the new ways).

The process starts with a trigger that highlights the need for change. At this point people involved in the change need to shed existing routines, beliefs, etc, in order to allow them to move forward (unfreezing). Change action plans are devised and following this the change occurs, which can be an unstable stage as the organisation is moving away from the familiar into the unknown. The final stage is known as refreeze. This is when the new system is fully accepted as the norm. If this stage is not reached, there is a risk of regression to the old system.

UNDERSTANDING THE IMPACT

In order to help manage and understand change it is essential to have an awareness of the impact that it can have upon individuals and groups.

Torrington et al. (1989, p. 106) identified that 'To some people, change means excitement and a thrill of being part of the action and keeping up with trends. For others, change feels like a threatening, imposed, dismantling of the stable order of things, with a great deal of uncertainty which is frightening.'

Upton and Brooks (1995) helped to analyse the impact of change upon an individual by identifying the nature of the human response and superimposing it onto the grief cycle outlined by Kubler-Ross in 1969 (see Example 3.2). The grief model can be very easily used to understand the reactions of people to the process of change.

It is important to note that any individual's reactions will vary in intensity and speed, and Upton and Brooks (1995) identified several factors affecting these responses:

■ Degree of choice or control.
■ How the person is affected by the change.
■ Previous experience of change.
■ Support available.

Example 3.2 indicates how this cycle could be applied in a scenario of someone's response to hospital closure.

Example 3.2

On being informed that the hospital where you work is closing in the next 2 years, you are initially shocked to hear the news. For a short while, whilst plans are being made, communications often reduce and there is a time of denial that anything will ever happen; you try not to think about it. As the reality begins to set in you become conscious that the closure is happening and may be angry and look for someone to blame. Your perceived level of competence to do anything about this is at its lowest when you realise you should have been looking for another job sooner and blame yourself for putting your head in the sand. If you stay in the post, being re-located by the Trust, you go though a period of adapting to the new situation. This is termed the bargaining stage, which can be unsettling but also challenging. The final stage of resolution commences when you start to work in the new hospital and realise it is not as bad as you thought it would be and it begins to feel like a secure environment again (internalisation).

Change can also have a significant effect on groups of people, particularly in their operational performance. Those people who work within teams will be aware that the efficiency and effectiveness is reliant upon each person performing as a team member and as an individual. In order for a team to function well members must be acquainted with each other and aware of everyone's roles and skills. When there are changes within the team, periods are required for re-adjustment. This is particularly noticeable when basic grades are on rotation or if locums are regularly used within a department. Tuckman (1965) described these within the 'Group Life Model'.

Tuckman proposed that groups go through a continual evolution process during team building and change. This process is evident whether a new team is being formed or if some members leave and are replaced. The first stage is referred to as 'forming'; when a group first meets they may be unaware of each other's roles, responsibilities and working patterns and may also have anxieties about the contribution they can make within the group. Once the group clarifies its role and begins to work on the issues concerned, members begin to assert their position and conflict is not uncommon ('storming'). In the next stage systems, processes and structures are analysed and people settle into their respective roles ('norming'). The performing stage is considered to be when people are functioning at their most effective. The final stage of 'mourning' takes place when the group ends or there is change in its membership. The cycle may then recommence.

Mark (1997) claims that certain factors may predict the team moving into another stage; these can be:

- Changes to team membership.
- Changes to task.
- Changes to environment.
- Changes to team norms or roles.

If the manager fails to acknowledge these issues during the change process, it could have a negative impact on the individual and the team.

Reflective questions:

- *Can you identify and consider an aspect of change that you have been part of?*
- *What was the impact of this change on yourself and your team?*

MANAGING CHANGE

For the early part of your working life, the likelihood is that your experience of change within the workplace will be largely one of imposed change rather than change you are personally instigating. There may be opportunities for you to initiate some changes within the department, however, and for this you need to be well prepared and have an awareness of the strategic intent.

French et al. (1985) identified eight specific components of successful change:

- Initial problem identification.
- Obtaining data.
- Problem diagnosis.
- Action planning.
- Implementation.
- Follow-up and stabilisation.

- Assessment of consequences.
- Learning from the process.

These components can be used as a checklist to assess if each step has been addressed. Problems are likely to arise if any component is omitted. The following section addresses these components under the headings of:

- Analysing the need for change.
- Planning and implementing change.
- Evaluating change.

Analysing the need for change

In order to assist your analysis of the changes required, an understanding of marketing strategies is invaluable. Marketing within the context of health and social care is about identifying the needs of the service user/organisation and analysing how your service might address them. In order to do this you must firstly analyse where your service fits into the organisation and wider context and then explore the core skills you/your profession/department possess.

So how might you analyse your service? One useful method is to use the instrument devised by the Boston Consulting Group (1970), known as the Growth Rate–Market Share Matrix or the Boston Matrix. This matrix can help you focus on those services that need development and investment, whilst ensuring that you are following the current trends (see Figure 3.4). Within this matrix there are four sections:

- 'Cash Cows' need low investment for high returns. These should be the core services of the organisation/department.
- 'Rising Stars' need high investment but will also provide high returns. These are usually the newer projects which have been instigated and are developing.
- 'A Problem Child' needs high investment but will only provide low returns. These are often new projects or 'craven dogs', which are taking much time and effort to organise but are not yet functioning effectively.

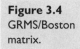

Figure 3.4
GRMS/Boston
matrix.

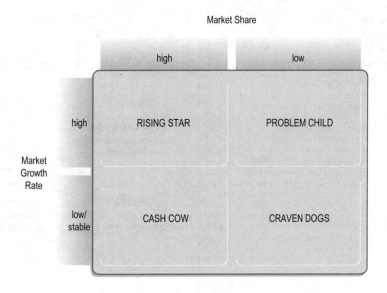

■ 'Craven Dogs' need low investment for low returns. These may be projects that have been running for many years and are no longer popular.

The concept is dynamic and suggests that through investment and effort aspects can be moved from one category to another so that a problem child can move to rising star to cash cow.

When analysing your service it is important to ensure you have at least one cash cow as this is going to represent the majority of your workload, and without it your service may fold. However, it is important to consider the life cycle of your cash cows because if they suddenly become superfluous to requirement, your service will seriously suffer. It is therefore important to develop your rising stars to replace those services once they reach the end of their life cycle. Those services that are in the rising stars category still require much investment but are providing rewards.

There may also be some services that you are hoping to nurture but are currently at the development stage. These fall into the problem child category as you will be investing much time in planning them; however, as they are not yet functioning you cannot rely on these to provide your main workload. Those services that are craven dogs either need massive investment to mobilise them into providing a viable service again or should be lost altogether. Although it does no harm to have one or two craven dogs a pack of them is likely to destroy your service and will create an unhealthy working environment for a practitioner. An example of how this can be applied for a service is highlighted in Figure 3.5.

Once at the stage of analysing specific aspects of the service there is an inclination to try to consider 'what else can I do/provide?'; however, it is often a good

Reflective questions:

■ *Can you formulate a matrix to identify and position your services/ aspects of your service on the grid?*
■ *What is the life cycle of your cash cows?*

Figure 3.5 Application of the GRMS/ Boston matrix – representing a re-ablement team running for 6 months.

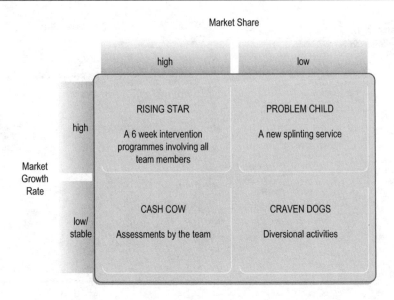

idea as a provider of services to separate what we *do* from what we *are for*. Recognising what purpose we fulfil helps us to think of things from the perspective of service users. Service users should not happen to want what we have; they should determine what we provide. It is difficult to meet people's expectations unless we endeavour to identify what they are. It is important to explore this thoroughly, as if data collected is incomplete or incorrect, the other stages are destined to fail. Due to the fast pace of change, this is very often the stage that people omit or undertake superficially, relying on personal judgement instead. Complete data will include both factual (legislation, evidence-based practice) and subjective information (impressions, fears). These can be explored by a variety of means to include questionnaires, satisfaction surveys, interviews and focus groups. When this data is collected it is important that you thoroughly analyse it in relation to the service and the organisation.

Within this stage it is important to consider all aspects of your service and the people who potentially require it. So how do you go about analysing this? Two tools that can be used to assist you are the PEST (as described above), and SWOT analyses.

When instigating change it is important to be aware of the external and internal forces, as these are likely to need addressing through the process of the change. A SWOT analysis considers these factors in relation to those that either drive or restrain the functioning of the organisation and divide them into four groups.

- *Strengths* or internal driving forces.
- *Weaknesses* or internal restraining forces.
- *Opportunities* or external driving forces.
- *Threats* or external restraining forces.

Identifying the internal forces (strengths and weaknesses) helps us to look at ourselves as an organisation and assess our ability to operate within the wider environment. Identifying the external forces (opportunities and threats) helps us to look outwards, thinking about our organisation in the context of this wider environment.

Often a matrix as illustrated in Figure 3.6 is used for the SWOT analysis and it is usually advisable to involve a range of people from the organisation in

Figure 3.6
Example of a SWOT analysis matrix.

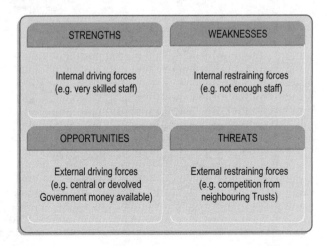

completing it (since perceptions can differ and others can bring new perspectives). The process of completing the matrix, therefore, is as important as the end result. In Figure 3.6 a single example for each section has been given; however, when undertaking your SWOT analysis you must fully consider and include all factors concerned as there are many pitfalls that people fall into when using this tool. These are:

- Omitting part of the grid.
- Confusing weaknesses and threats or strengths and opportunities.
- Mixing internal and external influences. Remember opportunities are *external* factors that provide you with options to help develop your service.
- Omitting key stakeholders' perspectives when looking at a service wide issue.
- Omitting key issues because they do not fit with your views.
- Not using the data collected to analyse and change the service. (Remember: completing the SWOT grid is only the first stage.)

Once the information is gathered using the SWOT grid, it must be analysed to help direct the change. In order to do this you must consider strategies to:

- Mobilise the driving forces.
- Overcome the restraining forces.

To mobilise the driving forces it is important to use them to your advantage – see also force field analysis above. This in turn will help to overcome the restraints. Working against policy decisions will be ineffective in allowing change of practice to progress smoothly. This is most easily explained by the use of a working example as shown in Figure 3.7.

Figure 3.7
Using a SWOT analysis.

You have undertaken an audit of staff documentation and it has become evident that the team are currently not meeting the standards that have been set. Your SWOT grid may resemble this:

STRENGTHS
Realistic standards already set
All members of staff have basic IT skills
Standardised documentation forms exist

WEAKNESSES
Not meeting standards
One old computer in department
Negative staff attitudes to paperwork
Staff carry very large caseloads

OPPORTUNITIES
Organisation keen to promote paperless offices
IT courses occurring within the organisation
Greater availability of a variety of IT resources
Government drive for evidence-based practice
Much evidence to support use of IT
Professional Code of Conduct
Money available for IT development

THREATS
Litigation
Professional Code of Conduct
Potential to be de-registered

To mobilise the driving forces your service could place a bid for the funding which is available in the organisation for IT development. To strengthen this bid you could utilise evidence-based practice both to support the purchase of additional IT and as investment, as it will serve not only to improve documentation, but also to find evidence to validate the intervention. Palm top computers are easily accessible by all members of the team, and if used by all staff could avoid duplication of written information. Accessing the training within the wider organisation will be a cost effective way to improve confidence and therefore compliance. Hence this has the potential to change staff attitudes about the time-consuming nature of documentation.

Planning and implementing change

Planning for change is vital and aims are essential. These must be carefully considered before implementing your plan and should be set and regularly reviewed. Iles (1997) highlighted that the benefits of planned change should be fully analysed and should outweigh the costs and risks if they are to be instigated. By undertaking this analysis a firm decision can then be made to start the change. Once this has been agreed a clear process needs to be devised.

At this stage it is also important to draw up a list of approximately 5–7 measurable critical success factors without which the project/service will fail (Austin 1997). These can later be used to evaluate the success of your project.

Below are examples of critical success factors for a new orthotics service:

- Appropriately skilled staff.
- Specific splinting equipment and materials.
- Inter-professional and inter-agency communication networks.
- Service users with specific splinting needs.
- Appropriate environmental resources, e.g. room, water, electricity.
- Effective documentation system.

It is important to highlight that certain skills are required to successfully instigate and lead change. Stewart (1997, p. 19) states that 'change, if it is to be successfully implemented must be managed'. This suggests that the process must be carefully planned. Malin et al. (2002, p. 91) believe it is everyone's responsibility to be involved in the process if it is to be successful, stating: 'Change is a task to be self-managed rather than a series of centrally driven restructurings: the focus is to create conditions, which require everyone to become a change-agent.'

It is in this early stage that there may also be resistance to change and conflict and the person instigating the change must address these issues. Blair (1993, p. 134) stated that 'as a manager, you need to solve or at least contain problems. Ignore them at your peril. If you deal with them, you can enhance the performance of the whole team.'

A key factor in instigating and managing change is motivation of staff. Hertzberg explored the theory of motivation in the 1950s presenting the 'Motivation Hygiene Theory' (Hertzberg 1968). This theory extended Maslow's 'Hierarchy of Needs' (Mullins 2002) and is more applicable to the work situation. The hygiene factors within a work environment are related to job context, e.g. job security, salary and terms and conditions. The motivational factors are related to the job content itself, i.e. recognition, nature of work, etc. Hertzberg stressed the need for managers to pay attention to the motivating factors as well as the hygiene factors.

It is well-documented that change produces anxiety as can be seen in earlier parts of this chapter; lack of information through the process can exacerbate this. Kanter (1989) in her entrepreneurial model and Plant (1987) both suggest that there will always be losers in the process of change; however, they also acknowledge the importance of analysing the extent of this loss before decisions are made, and ensuring that 'losers' are never dismissed.

Plant (1987, p. 46) stated that people managing change must 'communicate like you have never communicated before … anything that reduces uncertainty to an acceptable level will help.' Many years on this is still important; communication facilitators are now often used in projects to assist in the information dissemination process. These people are responsible for transferring information between departments and between levels, i.e. management to service. This role was also alluded to by Likert (1967) cited in Boss (1989) who referred to the importance of the linking-pins, or those people who simultaneously belong to two groups in an organisation. He outlined the linking-pin manager's role as reflecting the values, biases and opinions of each group, an essential role for change management.

Before the new project is released its potential success can be measured against the set criteria formulated during the planning stage. Austin (1997) describes this as critical success factor analysis. Earlier in the chapter an example of critical success factors were given for a specific project. If all these factors are evident then success of the project is viable. If one or more factors are missing then this ideally needs to be addressed prior to implementing the change.

Once the move has been made, it is important that sufficient time is given in which to allow the re-freezing stage to occur, providing that the new practice is safe. In the initial stages some resistance and conflict may still be present whilst people are familiarising themselves with the new work practice. During this early unstable period, evaluation of the success of the change may give inaccurate data.

Evaluating change

As with any service, new or old, it is essential to have mechanisms in place to control inputs and outputs. Within organisations there are usually government-controlled mechanisms like primary funding, those which are controlled centrally such as monthly statistic returns and finally departmental mechanisms such as analysis of the budget sheets and satisfaction surveys. These can similarly be employed to evaluate the success of your new development.

A change commitment grid is a useful way of analysing the effectiveness of the change management process and the extent to which opinion of key stakeholders has changed. An illustration of this can be seen in Figure 3.8 in relation to the development of a single assessment process.

The ability column indicates the level of influence that the various people within a department can have over a project. In the example the team manager has the greatest influence with the therapy assistant and secretary having the least. By analysing the totals of people changing their perspectives, a positive movement of staff commitment can be seen. This means that potentially the change has been managed successfully.

Figure 3.8
Change
commitment
grid – developing
a single
assessment
process.
Modified from
Kotler and
Schlesinger
(1979).

Stakeholders	Against	Passive	Facilitative	Drive	Ability
Team Manager				●▲	H
Deputies	●●	▲→		▲	M→H
Senior Therapist	●		▲		M
Junior Therapist		●	▲		M→L
Therapy Assistant	●▲				L
Secretary	●		▲		L
Total	5→1	1→1	0→3	1→2	

Key: ● Position at initial suggestion of proposed change

▲ Position concerning change at current time

Ability H = High   M = Medium   L = Low

At the evaluation stage the critical success factors can be utilised to guide the setting of specific criteria by which you can measure the effectiveness and quality of the new development.

Within the process of change there are always aspects that could be improved upon or could have been managed differently. Allied health professionals under the Health Professions Council have a responsibility for continuing professional development. It is therefore essential to reflect upon these aspects and document action learning points for the future.

ACCOMMODATING CHANGE AND REGAINING CONTROL

The earlier sections of this chapter have explored strategies to help instigate and manage change. This final part aims to assist you in making the change a positive experience for you.

Okay, so you have discovered that there are going to be major changes within your organisation. You have heard rumours about what these will entail and you know others do not agree with what is happening. What should you do?

Firstly, it is important to have all the facts. As within the therapeutic process, the importance of data gathering can never be underestimated. This is supported by Braverman and Fisher (1997) who emphasised the importance of being prepared for change by becoming fully informed. So what do you need to find out? The following guidelines and flow chart (Figure 3.9) will assist you in gaining the full picture and identify ways in which you can regain some control over the process.

Where has this change come from? Who is proposing it?

Determining this will allow you to analyse the level of control you are likely to be able to have. For example, if it is a new piece of legislation, you are wasting your energies trying to fight it. Although it is not advocated that you accept everything that comes your way, this type of change can only be fought at a much higher level and it is likely that the change will occur with or without your consent! If, however, this is a departmental initiative, you are likely to have more influence over its implementation. Factors driving change were highlighted earlier.

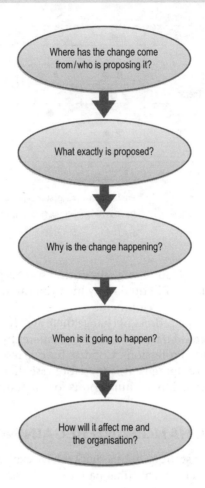

Figure 3.9
The change
exploration
process flow
chart.

What exactly is proposed?

Chinese whispers within an organisation can often result in serious inaccuracies in the information you have and on which you are basing your opinions. You do not have any right to influence policies and procedures when you have not taken the time to discover the facts. This information can be gained in many ways: it may be that your line manager can give you all the details (but ensure you know where their information has come from). Often with major changes, organisations will have discussion forums where you can hear about the proposals and ask questions, or consultation periods where you can submit your views for consideration.

Why is the change happening?

Change is often greeted by less resistance if the rationale behind it is understood Change often occurs from an internal influence, for example when a new manager is appointed. It may also happen in response to external factors, such as new legislation, threats from competitors or when service reviews indicate the need for improvement. Therefore, it is important that you take time to explore and understand the reason for the change.

When is it going to happen?

When there is constant change people feel that they do not have time to adjust to one practice before another is introduced. Ideally change should be planned and executed over an adequate period of time to allow for the full cycle of the process to be effective. However, sticking your head in the sand will not always slow the change down; a proactive approach is much more effective and could give you some control over the time element.

The change process has a macro- and a micro-effect and both need to be considered.

How will it affect the organisation/department? – the macro level

It is important to consider these details. If you know how something is likely to affect your organisation or your managers, you are likely to have a much greater understanding of the wider issues involved and will be better informed to test and question the proposals, which is equally important (Correia and Volger 1993). Adopting an objective perspective will allow you to present any ideas or opinions professionally, therefore increasing your credibility within your department or organisation. This will be particularly useful in future situations.

How will it affect me? – the micro level

Once you have established an objective baseline, you must think about how the change is likely to affect you. This may indicate the reasons for your concerns and also give you a focus for your potential influence, particularly if the issue is very important to you. For example, rather than fight re-location to new premises because parking in the area will be very difficult for you, try to find out if there are any ways that parking might be addressed.

If each of these aspects is considered and understood you are automatically in a position of greater control and the process of change is likely to be a less stressful experience. You never know, you might just enjoy it!

CONCLUSION

This chapter has illustrated the dynamic nature of change and the importance of maintaining the momentum. It has demonstrated the need to acknowledge that this is an aspect of your working life that is very difficult/impossible to stop, but that there are many chances to influence it.

The data gathering stage is especially important and the analysis of the need for change must be undertaken thoroughly. The tools identified throughout this chapter should assist you in this process.

Emphasis is placed on the importance of thorough preparation and open communication, to encourage the success of the change, which should be a carefully staged process.

Now that you have read the chapter try to answer the questions below to help you to consolidate your understanding of the change process.

Reflective questions:

- Consider a situation involving change within your workplace. In light of the information presented in this chapter, what reflections can you make on the positive and negative aspects of this change?
- Can you use one of the marketing tools in this chapter to analyse an aspect of your service that you consider needs reviewing?
- Can you develop this analysis to highlight at least three areas that may benefit from change and outline a strategy to support this?
- In addition to your practice skills, can you analyse different knowledge and skills you might already have and those you still need to refine/develop to be effective within the organisation?

REFERENCES

Austin N 1997 Strategic planning. In: Austin N, Dopson S (eds). *The clinical directorate.* Radcliffe Medical Press, Oxford, pp. 77–100.

Blair GM 1993 *Starting to manage – the essential skills.* Chartwell Bratt, Bromley.

Boss RW 1989 *Organisational development in healthcare.* Addison-Wesley Publishing Company, New York.

Boston Consulting Group 1970 *Product Portfolio Matrix.* pp. 1–313. Online. Available: http://64.58.136/search/cache?p = boston + consulting + group 16 May 2003.

Braverman B, Fisher G 1997 Managing care: survival skills for the future. *Occupational Therapy in Healthcare* 10: 13–31.

Cameron A, Masterson A 1998 The changing policy context of occupational therapy in emerging systems of the 21st century. *American Journal of Occupational Therapy* 61: 556–560.

Correia S, Volger J 1993 Patient focused care. *British Journal of Occupational Therapy* 56: 107.

French WL, Kast FE, Rosenzweig JE 1985 *Understanding human behaviour in organisations.* Harper and Rowe, London.

Hamer S, Collinson G 1999 *Achieving evidence-based practice. A handbook for practitioners.* Bailliere Tindall, London.

Hertzberg F 1968 'One more time: how do you motivate employees?' *Harvard Business Review* 46: 53–62.

Iles V 1997 *Really managing healthcare.* Open University Press, Buckingham.

Kanter RM 1989 *When giants learn to dance.* Unwin, London.

Kotler J, Schlesinger L 1979 *Choosing strategies for change. Harvard Business Review* 57(2): 106–114.

Kubler-Ross E 1969 On death and dying. Routledge, London.

Lewin K 1958 Group decisions and social change. In: Maccoby E, Newcomb T, Hartley E (eds). *Readings in social psychology.* Methuen, London.

Lloyd C, King R 2002 Organisational change and occupational therapy. *British Journal of Occupational Therapy* 65(12): 536–542.

Lloyd C, Bassett H, King R 2002 Mental health: how well are occupational therapists equipped for a changed practice environment? *Australian Journal of Occupational Therapy* 49:163–166.

Malin N, Wilmot S, Manthorpe J 2002 *Key concepts and debates in health and social policy.* Open University Press, Buckingham.

Mark A 1997 Working in teams. In: Austin N, Dopson S (eds). *The clinical directorate.* Oxford, Radcliffe Medical Press, pp. 1–16.

Mullins LJ 2002 *Management and organisational behaviour,* 6th edn. Prentice Hall, Harlow.

Plant R 1987 *Managing change and making it stick.* Fontana Paperbacks, London.

Shervington M 2003 *A CaN HeLP approach to change*, pp. 1–2.
Online. Available:
www.john.semour-associates.co.uk/helpapproachspreadlow.pdf
15 May 2003.
Stewart A 1997 Communication, promotion and marketing in occupational therapy. *British Journal of Therapy and Rehabilitation* 4(4): 68–69.
Torrington D, Weightman J, Johns K 1989 *Effective management – people and organisation*. Prentice Hall International (UK), Hertfordshire.
Tuckman BW 1965 Development sequence in small groups. *Psychological Bulletin* 63: 384–399.
Upton T, Brooks B 1995 *Managing change in the NHS*. Kogan Page, London.

RECOMMENDED READING

Decker D 1995 Market testing – does it bring home the bacon? *Health Service Journal* 19th January, pp. 26–28.
Finnegan M 1997 Marketing occupational therapy: Can we do it? *British Journal of Therapy and Rehabilitation* 4(4): 195–199.
Gann N 1996 *Managing change in voluntary organisations – a guide to practice*. Open University Press, Buckingham.
Henry J, Mayle D (eds) 2002 *Managing innovation and change*, 2nd edn. Sage, London.
Jacobs K, Logigian MK 1999 *Functions of a manager in occupational therapy*, 3rd edn. Slack, New Jersey.
Martin V 2003 *Leading change in health and social care*. Routledge, London.
Swage T 2000 *Clinical governance in healthcare practice*. Butterworth Heinemann, Oxford.

PART 1 Setting the scene for practice

Conclusion

Lyn Westcott and Teena J. Clouston

This first part of the book has looked at some key areas that help you to understand the bigger picture in which an individual practises. The context of health and social care (Chapter 1) is important to understand as an AHP because your experience of practice will always be shaped by and sited within a wider health and social care agenda. This is true whether you are employed by statutory services, the voluntary sector or even private practice.

Systems-thinking (Chapter 2) may have been a new concept to you but its relevance for AHP practitioners in health and social care should now be much clearer to appreciate. Although you may not have realised that you work within a system or sub-system, understanding this concept is vital to make sense of how teams, organisations and societies function.

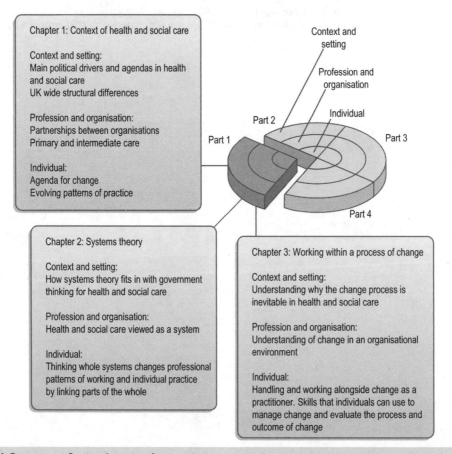

Chapter 1: Context of health and social care

Context and setting:
Main political drivers and agendas in health and social care
UK wide structural differences

Profession and organisation:
Partnerships between organisations
Primary and intermediate care

Individual:
Agenda for change
Evolving patterns of practice

Context and setting

Profession and organisation

Individual

Part 1
Part 2
Part 3
Part 4

Chapter 2: Systems theory

Context and setting:
How systems theory fits in with government thinking for health and social care

Profession and organisation:
Health and social care viewed as a system

Individual:
Thinking whole systems changes professional patterns of working and individual practice by linking parts of the whole

Chapter 3: Working within a process of change

Context and setting:
Understanding why the change process is inevitable in health and social care

Profession and organisation:
Understanding of change in an organisational environment

Individual:
Handling and working alongside change as a practitioner. Skills that individuals can use to manage change and evaluate the process and outcome of change

Part 1 Summary Setting the scene for practice

Working within a process of change (Chapter 3) has highlighted a key area that practitioners and organisations may find difficult to accommodate. However, successful recognition and assimilation of the processes of change within your work can enable AHP practitioners to provide effective quality services that are responsive to need.

The figure provides a brief summary of key issues considered throughout Part 1, highlighting their relevance to individual practitioners, the professions and organisations in which they work, together with the context and settings of practice.

PART 2 Development of the professions and individual practitioner

Introduction

Lyn Westcott and Teena J. Clouston

The second part of the book sets out to examine some key areas that will help you understand the professional dimensions in which an individual practises. These areas are:

- Understanding health and social care professions from sociological perspectives (Chapter 4).
- Thinking about teamworking and collaboration (Chapter 5).
- Continuing professional development (Chapter 6).
- Aspects of professionalism (Chapter 7).

As an individual allied health professional (AHP), you need to understand what it means to be a practitioner and a registered member of your own unique profession. You also need to consider the role that you fulfil in a team situation and how this is shaped by both your professional and individual identity. Part of this role is demonstrating your ability to develop your practice continuously to meet the ever-changing needs of your profession and organisation. In this part of the book, these issues are examined with a more individual and profession-based focus than in previous chapters. However, contextual factors such as guiding legislation and key drivers for change are highlighted to help you link professional considerations with the wider agenda for health and social care in the UK. In order to make sense of Part 2, you are advised to bear in mind the three domains of context and setting, profession and organisation and also individual practice. This will help you understand why the text is relevant to you. These themes are revisited within the conclusion and summary found at the end of Part 2, which includes an illustration of key areas within each chapter under these headings.

4 Understanding healthcare professions from sociological perspectives

Steven W. Whitcombe

> **LEARNING OUTCOMES**
>
> Following this chapter the reader should be able to:
> - Identify different sociological perspectives regarding the study of professions.
> - Apply sociological theories to explain the 'professionalisation' of health and social care occupations.
> - Examine the influence of contemporary health and social care policy on the current and future practice of allied health professionals.

INTRODUCTION

The concept of a professional occupation may mean different things to different people; for example an expectation of quality, work that requires specialist skills, or more simply a job that is paid. This chapter draws on sociological perspectives to define and explain professionalism within the context of the UK health and social care system. In particular the chapter will explore the relatively new professionalisation of allied healthcare practitioners such as occupational therapists, physiotherapists and radiographers.

Why explore the subject of professions from sociological perspectives?

Sociology is the study of how the society in which we live influences our everyday behaviour, our attitudes to life and our cultural pursuits. Sociology is also the study of how we, as human beings shape the society to which we belong. A sociological understanding of life events requires the individual to take 'a step back' from their everyday situation and look at the world in a fresh light. In regard to the study of professions this may involve not accepting the notion of professions at face value and the posing of such questions as:

- What is a profession?
- What is the purpose of professions and how do they evolve?
- How can we account for the differences in terms of power and status between different 'so called' professional groups?

Whilst sociologists tend to agree on the importance of studying human society, they often disagree on how to go about studying society, how to account for the various forms that societies take and how to interpret the influence of societies on human behaviour. This chapter looks at different sociological arguments concerning the nature of professions in an attempt to answer the questions posed above. It also provides you with a sociological framework to ask the same questions (and other questions that follow) of the profession to which you belong. It thus offers you a 'social lens' to reflect upon how your professional role and your relationship with other health/social care professions impact upon the service you deliver.

PROFESSIONS – A TAXONOMIC DEFINITION

The taxonomic or trait approach of characterising a profession was popular amongst sociologists up until the 1960s. This consisted of defining a profession according to a list of special features they possessed. Typically these included the following:

■ Possession of a specialised body of knowledge and skills.
■ Freedom and autonomy to regulate practice.
■ An extensive period of education and training before members are permitted to practise.
■ A code of conduct that governs practice.
   (Modified from Gomm 1996.)

The trait approach is useful in terms of comparing professional groups with one another in order to identify what features they do and do not share, but it offers little insight into how professions attain these characteristics in the first place (Blane 1997, Jones and Stewart 1998).

Reflective questions:

■ *To what extent does your profession possess all the features listed above?*
■ *How do the features your profession has compare with other health and social care professions?*

PROFESSIONS – A FUNCTIONALIST POSITION

The functionalist view of the nature of professions (similarly to the taxonomic/trait approach) was popular with many sociologists up to the middle of the twentieth century. Functionalists hold the view that society is made of up of inter-related parts or systems, for example, religion, the educational system, the family, etc. that work together to produce a common social order. Classical functionalist sociologists include Auguste Comte (1798–1857) and Emile Durkheim (1858–1917) who argued that society is held together by a moral consensus, i.e. a culture consisting of shared values and acceptable behaviours (norms). Children or individuals new to society learn these shared values and cultural norms through a process known as socialisation (Giddens 2001).

From a functionalist perspective, professions exist to serve society; their work is deemed as being of 'functional relevance' to the social system. The period of training/education necessary in order to acquire professional status is rewarded with certain freedoms and privileges such as better working conditions and higher pay than other occupations. Furthermore, the professions' right to self-regulation and control is given by society on the basis that they do not take advantage of their privileged position through using their esoteric knowledge in an exploitative manner.

More recently in the UK and the USA, functionalist theory has lost favour amongst sociologists and has been criticised on a number of grounds. First, functionalism tends to present an 'over-socialised' view of humankind; an emphasis on social structures and the agencies of socialisation (e.g. family, work) that overshadows individual human action, creativity and choice. Second, functionalists, through stressing social cohesion, do not adequately account for social change within society. Indeed, functionalism suggests societies evolve over time and changes in the social system arise for the good of all, out of societal need. However, this argument does not account for less harmonious, rapid or sudden social change that can result in new social and political structures, for example, the fall of the communist states in Eastern Europe (Jones 2003). Third, functionalists argue that societies work on the basis of a common consensus, and tend to overlook discord between individuals, or groups of people in society. As Jones and Stewart (1998) point out, if all professions share common values and a sense of public altruism, why do conflicts occur between different healthcare professions?

Reflective question:

Consider your own experiences of professional conflict. What were the underlying causes and how could/can this be resolved?

PROFESSIONS – A MARXIST POSITION

Karl Marx (1818–1883) was a philosopher, historian and sociologist who was interested in the development of a capitalist society. Capitalism refers to an economic system where goods and services are mass produced and sold to a wide range of consumers. For Marx, capitalist society consisted of two broad groups of people: those who owned the means of production (e.g. factory owners), whom he termed the bourgeoisie, and the working class known as the proletariat, who sold their labour to the bourgeoisie. Marx argued that capitalist society is fraught with tension because ownership of the means of production allows the bourgeoisie to exploit the proletariat and therefore remain in a wealthy position at the expense of the much poorer working class. Unlike functionalist theory then, Marx advocated a society governed by structural conflict arising from economic difference between classes, rather than a society driven by cultural consensus.

Writers influenced by Marx, such as Navarro (1986) argue that the role of healthcare professions is to act as well-paid agents of the bourgeoisie and uphold the capitalist system. Although there are differences between healthcare professional groups in terms of status and power, this is accounted for by their relative importance to the bourgeoisie. Marxists maintain that healthcare workers assist the capitalist state through encouraging workers to seek a biomedical reason for all ill health, which detracts from the real causes of most ill health, i.e. social and economic disadvantage.

One criticism levelled at Marxism is that too much weight is given to the idea that human action is largely economically motivated. Also, as Nettleton (1995) notes: Marxists tend to ignore the fact that service users do not necessarily accept medical/health professional interpretations concerning the causation of illness.

PROFESSIONS – A SOCIAL ACTION POSITION

Most recently, social action theories have tended to take precedence over both functionalist and Marxist arguments within the sociology of professions. Social action perspectives are influenced by the work of Max Weber (1864–1920) who, unlike Durkheim and Marx, was more interested in the action or behaviours of people in society rather than social structures (e.g. class). Weber believed the ideas and motivation of people engendered social change. Whilst he acknowledged the importance of social structures in constraining human behaviour, Weber argued that people are essentially free to make sense of, or interpret their own social circumstances and behave in ways that they choose. Furthermore, Weber believed people choose to act in certain ways to achieve the ends they desire (Jones 2003).

Following on from Weber, theorists such as Parkin (1979) have looked at how groups of people acquire professional status and maintain their place in society. Key to this is the concept of social closure, i.e. how occupational groups are able to take advantage of social and economic circumstances to gain a position of power, then monopolise this position through restricting entry to the profession and area of work. The rise of the medical profession is often cited by action theorists to illustrate the idea of social closure because it developed in the midst of social change within British and European society that sociologists refer to as 'modernity'. This is characterised by the industrial age (i.e. the rise of capitalism), that generated changing work patterns, centralised forms of government and set in motion an acceptance of a scientific or rational view of the world rather than a dependence on traditional religious explanations.

Saks (1998) points out that medical practitioners in the nineteenth century (surgeons, physicians and apothecary surgeons) gained a stronghold in the provision of healthcare from uniting together to form the single occupational group, i.e. 'doctors' legitimised by the 1858 Medical Registration Act. This Act created the General Medical Council and allowed doctors to become the first healthcare profession to attain self-regulatory powers and control over their education, training and admission. By the twentieth century, the medical position was further strengthened by modern society's growing affinity with the scientific and biomedical model. As the search for the biological basis of disease gathered speed, doctors were placed more and more in the position of 'expert' able to exercise control over a deferential and lay public.

Action theorists point out that other healthcare occupations seeking professional status and all that entails, e.g. autonomy over their own affairs, are disadvantaged because they have to convince both the state (government) of their right to professional status and an established medical profession which will endeavour to protect its own interests. Healthcare practitioners such as dentists and optometrists have perhaps been most successful in gaining professional status outside that of medicine, but at the cost of limiting their expertise to parts of the body.

The social action approach, more so than any other approach regarding the study of professions, acknowledges the behaviours of individuals (or groups of people) in gaining a professional identity. In doing so, however, social action theorists can be criticised for presenting an image of healthcare professionals as essentially self-serving rather than reflecting the public interest.

THE PROFESSIONALISATION OF ALLIED HEALTH WORKERS

Historically, allied health professionals (AHPs) have not had the status and powers to control their own affairs to the extent that the medical profession has achieved. Explanations for the relative lack of autonomy of allied health workers differ, depending upon the sociological school of thought. Functionalists would suggest that AHPs, in common with nursing, lack a distinct specialised knowledge base and depend on medicine in this respect. In consequence, both nursing and AHPs require a shorter period of training than doctors. The medical profession, on the other hand, has a stronger part to play in the eradication of disease than AHPs and the importance of this function is rewarded in terms of greater freedom and higher remuneration.

Marxist sociologists have a different view. They propose that AHPs are not as important to the ruling class as the medical profession in regard to perpetuating the idea that illness/disease is arbitrary rather than a nexus to the working conditions of the capitalist state. Thus, the medical profession is allowed more authority in terms of governing their working practices than AHPs because they play a more significant ideological role in upholding bourgeois hegemony. Finally, as outlined above, social action theorists account for the difference in autonomy and status of the medical profession compared to AHPs by focusing on the medical profession's success in developing a dominant position in the provision of healthcare since the nineteenth century.

Their relative lack of status aside, however, there has been an increasing trend towards the professionalisation of AHPs over the latter half of the twentieth century. This has been accelerated by a changing view of health in the UK caused by a gradual decline in the incidence of infectious diseases such as tuberculosis and an increase in the rate of long-term chronic conditions such as cancer and heart disease. Furthermore, people in the western world today can expect, on average, to live longer than their ancestors. The causes of disease and ill health are now recognised to be complex involving social, psychological and environmental influences as well as biological/chemical factors. Changing patterns of disease coupled with the move from a biomedical model to a holistic view of health necessitates a pluralistic health service with an increasingly specialised workforce. AHPs have responded to the changing perception of health and disease by expanding their skills and in some respects developing a systematic knowledge base independent of medicine. For example, occupational therapists have begun to produce their own theories regarding the relationship of occupation to health. Since the 1990s entry level educational programmes to the professions of physiotherapy, occupational therapy and radiography have changed from diploma to degree and it is now possible to gain Masters and doctoral qualifications in allied health subjects. The growing research culture within the allied health professions has been assisted by setting up, or in some cases relocating professional programmes within the university sector with access to wider resources than those generally available in isolated training schools.

Paradoxically, the professionalisation of AHPs has gained ground at a time when the autonomy of the medical profession has been attacked from at least three fronts. First, successive government reforms to the provision of healthcare has created stronger managerial control of services which has, in effect, curbed medical power (Dingwall 1996). This began with reforms introduced by the

Conservative Government in the 1980s and with legislation such as The National Health Service and Community Care Act (1990) that brought about the internal market and the purchaser/provider split. The intention of the internal market was to address the problems of competing healthcare demands on constrained resources. Purchasers of health services, e.g. general practitioners, were given budgets to buy healthcare from providers, e.g. hospitals. This meant the providers of services were in competition with each other and medical interventions came under of the close scrutiny of hospital managers in an attempt to cut costs and deliver economically viable services.

Second, over recent years, service users (and users' organisations such as SANE) have been much more proactive in expressing their health and social needs, although this does not necessarily equate with what is offered from the medical community (Morgan 1993). However, the rights of service users have been endorsed by the legislation above, designed to give more power to the consumer and the opportunity to complain when they don't get the services they require.

Third, people are generally now more aware of health-related issues, through increased media coverage and ease of access to information from electronic sources such as the internet. An evolving lay knowledge of health topics has encouraged some sociologists to propose that medicine is becoming 'de-professionalised'. This suggests that an increased public awareness of medical knowledge challenges the authority of doctors and as such the power imbalance of the 'expert' medical professional and the 'non-expert' patient is re-addressed.

Also, the authority of doctors has been challenged through the exposition of fallible medical practices, for example, the case of Harold Shipman. Such pernicious practice increasingly places scientific/medical knowledge under inspection from people living in what contemporary sociologists like Ulrich Beck (1992) and Anthony Giddens (1999) refer to as a 'risk society'. For both Beck and Giddens the advent of modernity brought about fairly stable ways of living, job security and a trust in the scientific paradigm. Today however, a large decline in the western manufacturing industry and the rise of the service sector has led to shifting employment patterns and greater personal instability for people at both an economic and social level. Modern society or 'late modernity' is also characterised by distrust in the certainty of science. Science is now more than ever open to question; disagreements between scientists and indeed, about the nature of knowledge itself is given over to the public domain. Modern society creates risk; risk in whom to trust and in whom to believe, which expert is right and which expert is wrong. A risk society is also a society full of choice, e.g. choice about how to treat illness and about whom to consult; ultimately more choice means more decisions. Despite blows to the autonomy of the medical profession however, it is still fair to suggest that public faith in the virtues of the medical model remains intact.

ALLIED HEALTH PROFESSIONS AND CURRENT HEALTHCARE REFORM

The election of the Labour Government in 1997 faced two key issues with regard to the running of the National Health Service (NHS). First, there was a need to take account of the rising assertiveness of consumers, i.e. the general public, in expressing their needs and wants from the Health Service and appease any trace of public anxiety concerning falling standards of healthcare. Second, the New

Labour Government, like the Conservative Government it replaced was faced with high demands on health services with limited staff, resources and money available to pay for them. Labour's response was to produce strategies and legislation designed to produce flexibility in terms of service delivery but at the same time to have a clear focus on the quality of health services. This 'modernisation' agenda was designed to place the service user at the centre of health provision, give more control to the front line staff delivering health services (and less control to hospital managers), whilst at the same time introducing quality initiatives such as clinical governance. These strategies were produced in part, to protect the service user from unscrupulous practitioners. One of the key structural changes to the NHS introduced by Labour was the abolition of the competitive internal market and NHS Trusts. New primary care trusts (PCTs) have been created in England (local health boards in Wales, NHS boards in Scotland and health and social services boards in Northern Ireland) with the responsibility for both planning and delivery of health services for local populations. A key function of the PCTs and their regional equivalents is to lead the way in the integration of health and social services through developing shared working practices and greater co-operation between professionals working within different organisations, the goal being to provide the service user with a 'seamless service'.

The modernisation agenda has a number of consequences for the working practices of the allied health professions and professionals. The NHS Plan: A Plan for Investment, A Plan for Reform (DoH 2000a), calls for the greater use of care protocols to determine how common health conditions should be treated. Protocol-based care is designed to make best use of available skills regardless of professional background and by so doing actively encourages crossing of traditional health/social care professional boundaries. The 'New' Labour Government proposed that by 2004 the majority of NHS staff would be working under agreed protocols that encourage the flexible application of scarce.resources.

Meeting the Challenge: A Strategy for the Allied Health Professions (DoH 2000b) sets out the role(s) open to AHPs with regard to the implementation and delivery of care protocols. The strategy advocates that AHPs extend their professional roles to fully embrace the notion of flexible working. Examples of extended roles cited by Meeting the Challenge, include podiatrists specialising in foot surgery techniques, dieticians monitoring blood and adjusting insulin, and radiographers (in breast cancer services) reading mammograms. In August 2003 a Department of Health press release proposed 10 key roles for the AHPs designed to help practitioners improve patient care and build upon the suggestions of extended role outlined in the NHS Plan (2000a) and Meeting the Challenge (2000b). The roles, which were developed with representatives from all AHPs, include the opportunity for practitioners to be the first point of contact for patient care, to manage and lead teams, and to take an active role in strategic planning and policy development; and for AHPs (working with protocols) the opportunity to diagnose, request and assess diagnostic tests and prescribe medication. This builds on, for example, the role of physiotherapists, who already have the right to prescribe medication to patients under patient group directives, i.e. via plans devised in consultation with doctors.

Meeting the Challenge (DoH 2000b) sets out changes to the way health/social care professionals are trained proposing a stronger emphasis on inter-professional education at undergraduate/pre-registration level with common foundation programmes that give students the chance to switch careers and training paths more easily. One example of inter-professional learning is the New Generation Project at Southampton University in collaboration with the University of Portsmouth and Isle of Wight NHS Workforce Development Confederation. This project focuses on implementing a programme of common learning for students entering 11 different health and social care professions and encourages students to think about issues such as role blurring and develop skills in team-working and multi-disciplinary problem solving (College of Occupational Therapists 2003).

A further proposal within the Meeting the Challenge (DoH 2000b) strategy is the introduction by 2004 of 'therapist consultant' posts that provide new opportunities for AHPs to advance their careers. Consultant AHPs will be expected to form care protocols with senior medical and nursing colleagues as well as retaining an 'expert' clinical role. Together with demonstrating expert practice, the core functions of AHP consultants should include professional leadership, the provision of education and training opportunities for their colleagues, the practice of research and the facilitation of service evaluation.

In recognition of the additional responsibilities and skills required of healthcare workers who wish to take up consultant posts or extend their professional roles, the Government has modernised the pay system for NHS staff (see Chapter 1). Under 'Agenda for Change' there is one set of terms and conditions which apply to all staff groups and a single pay spine divided into eight bands (eight being the highest) for nurses, AHPs and other healthcare workers, the intention being to reward staff on the basis of what they do rather than on their professional title (Unison 2003). The new pay system is also designed to permit easier career progression for support staff, e.g. physiotherapy assistants with a desire to adopt new roles and/or extra duties. Advancement through the new pay structure will depend upon all staff demonstrating they possess the necessary abilities for a particular post. A knowledge and skills framework (KSF) will be used to determine the starting point for staff on the pay structure and through the process of annual developmental review the KSF will be also be used to support staff claims for promotion, or movement into a higher pay band.

In tandem with the move to generate flexibility in the delivery of health services the Government is also committed to improving the quality of services by modernising systems of professional regulation. The Health Act 1999 proposed the replacement of the Council for Professions Supplementary to Medicine (CPSM) with a new, smaller and more unified regulative body for allied health professionals, i.e. The Health Professions Council (HPC). The HPC was established in 2001 and has been in operation since April 2002. The HPC is charged with the responsibility for setting and monitoring standards for professional training and conduct. Currently representing 13 occupational groups the Council has the authority to regulate other staff groups in the future providing they meet the standards set for its existing members. The HPC has a strong lay representative and has greater powers than the previous body (CPSM) to deal with individual professionals who pose an unacceptable risk to service users. Since July 2003 professionals registered with the Council have protection of title and there are plans in the future to link registration with evidence of continuing professional development (see Chapter 6).

> **Reflective questions:**
>
> *What do you think about the new extended roles proposed for AHPs? How do you feel, for example about the prospect of you or your colleagues being able to prescribe medication?*

ALLIED HEALTH PROFESSIONS AND THE FUTURE

The healthcare plans introduced by New Labour clearly create opportunities for AHPs to extend their roles and develop skills and as a result improve professional status. However, the move toward AHPs implementing extended roles does heighten some concerns about protection of both the professional and the service user. Mounce et al. (2001) argue, for example, that the College of Occupational Therapists and the Chartered Society of Physiotherapy have both identified a range of concerns around the supervision of therapists undertaking extended duties and issues around professional accountability and indemnity which has yet to be resolved. Allied health workers undertaking extended roles need to be aware that some of these new practices may not be covered by their normal professional insurance.

Furthermore, opportunities for professional development, whilst attractive to the individual health practitioner, may present a threat to the survival of the profession to which the individual belongs. Historically the professional training of allied health workers is based upon exclusivity and a move towards extended roles together with the expansion of initiatives such as inter-professional training 'muddies the waters' and may heighten worries among AHPs about the rise of generic working, and ultimately the birth of generic therapists. If however, professionals serve the needs of society, then it could be argued that the erosion of distinct professional groups is largely unimportant. Surely, what matters is that health/social professionals possess the skills needed by society regardless of professional title?

What is clear is that the needs of society are subject to change and therefore survival of a healthcare profession depends upon its ability to adapt to meet the needs of a dynamic world. Giddens (1999) argues that modern society demands individuals to constantly remould themselves to cope with the changing pace of life. Late modernity is less grounded in tradition and established ways of living than previous societies, requiring people to adjust more quickly to their changing surroundings, a process that Giddens refers to as social reflexivity. As AHPs become more professionalised and expand their repertoire of skills perhaps they also need to embrace this process of reflexivity. Allied professionals need to engage in a dialogue between themselves about what skills they share and where their practices and skills differ, and moreover, what healthcare consumers need and who is best placed to provide it. The AHPs' willingness or reluctance to honestly consider such questions returns us to the sociological perspectives outlined at the beginning of this chapter in an attempt to answer the more fundamental question of whose interests health professionals really serve.

SUMMARY

This chapter has considered different sociological arguments on the nature and purpose of professions. It has explored the 'professionalisation' of allied health workers at a time where the autonomy of established professions such as medicine has been challenged by the notion of consumerism and increased public awareness of health-related issues.

In the current economic and political climate it is unlikely that AHPs will ever attain the same powers to control their own affairs that were given or gained (depending on your point of view) by the medical profession.

The future of healthcare provision does provide the opportunity for practitioners to develop their skills, and more than ever before work beyond their traditional boundaries. Whether such developments are likely to improve services and address service users' needs or create tensions and 'turf battles' between different professional providers remains to be seen.

Reflective questions:

■ *Whose interests do you think allied healthcare professionals serve – their own, consumers' or both?*
■ *Do professional boundaries really matter?*
■ *What do you think the future holds for health/social care practitioners?*

REFERENCES

Beck U 1992 *Risk society: towards a new modernity.* Sage, London.

Blane D 1997 Health professions. In: Scambler G (ed.) *Sociology as applied to medicine,* 4th edn. WB Saunders, London, pp. 212–224.

College of Occupational Therapists 2003 Learning together to work together. *Occupational Therapy News* 11(5): 17–18.

Department of Health 2000a *The NHS Plan: a plan for investment, a plan for reform.* HMSO, London.

Department of Health 2000b *Meeting the Challenge: a strategy for the allied health professions.* HMSO, London.

Department of Health 2003 Press Release: *Allied health professionals receive tools to improve patient care,* 14 August 2003.
Online. Available:
http://www.info.doh.gov.uk/intpress.nsf/page/2003-0308
27 August 2003.

Dingwall R 1996 Professions and social order in a global society. Plenary paper for the ISA Working Group Conference, University of Nottingham.

Giddens A 1999 *Runaway world: how globalisation is reshaping our lives.* Profile Books, London.

Giddens A 2001 *Sociology,* 4th edn. Polity, Cambridge.

Gomm R 1996 Professions and professionalism. In: Aitken V, Jellicoe H (eds). *Behavioural science for health professionals.* Macmillan, London.

Jones P 2003 *Introducing social theory.* Polity, Cambridge.

Jones RK, Stewart A 1998 The sociology of the health professions. In: Jones D, Blair SEE, Hartery T et al. (eds). *Sociology and occupational therapy, an integrated approach.* Churchill Livingstone, Edinburgh, pp. 131–142.

Morgan S 1993 *Community mental health: practical approaches to long-term problems.* Chapman and Hall, London.

Mounce K, Ryan S, Cushnaghan et al. 2001 Planned national changes to allied health professional career structures. In: Carr A (ed.) *Defining the extended clinical role for allied health professionals in rheumatology.* Arthritis Research Campaign, Derbyshire.

Navarro V 1986 *Crisis health and medicine: a social critique.* Tavistock, London.

Nettleton S 1995 *The sociology of health and illness.* Polity, Cambridge.

Parkin F 1979 *Marxism and class theory: a bourgeois critique.* Tavistock, London.
Saks M 1998 Professionalism and health care. In: Field D, Taylor S (eds). *Sociological perspectives on health, illness and health care.* Blackwell Science, London, pp. 174–192.
The NHS and Community Care Act 1990. HMSO, London.
The Health Act 1999. HMSO, London.
Unison 2003 *Agenda for change: a summary.* Unison, London.

RECOMMENDED READING

Gomm R 1996 Professions and professionalism. In: Aitken V, Jellicoe H (eds). *Behavioural science for health professionals.* Macmillan, London.

* Although a little dated in parts, offers some good learning activities relevant to all allied health professionals.

Jones P 2003 *Introducing social theory.* Polity Press, Cambridge.

* An excellent starter for those new to the subject of sociology. The book impressively addresses both classical and contemporary social theorists in a very readable format.

Jones D, Stewart A 1998 The sociology of the health professions. In: Jones D et al. (eds). Sociology and occupational therapy. an integrated approach. Churchill Livingstone, Edinburgh.

* Introduces the idea of a relationship between professional status and gender, a concept which was not considered in this chapter. Like Gomm's chapter cited above, Jones and Stewart also provide good examples of learning activities that are related to occupational therapy practice but which can be applied to all AHPs.

Thinking about teamworking and collaboration

Paul K. Wilby

LEARNING OUTCOMES

This chapter aims to enable you:
- To gain an understanding of the concept of teamworking.
- To be able to consider your role in a team.
- To identify the common goals shared by your team and the 'inches' (the small steps and compromises) that are needed to achieve them.

INTRODUCTION

Teamworking has always been an important issue in health and social care. Terms such as joined up working, multi-professional teamworking, collaborative working and working in partnerships have been used to attempt to try and encapsulate the importance of delivering services in this way. The present modernisation in health and social care incorporates the partnership agenda which emphasises integration at organisational, professional and team levels. Further, documents such as Shifting the Balance of Power (Department of Health (DoH) 2001 and 2002) promote inclusion of the service user as an active member of the health and social care team. The overall vision of this integrated and inclusive teamworking is effective, high quality service delivery. However, in order for that to be realised different ways of working need to be utilised and this has fundamental repercussions on teams and the individuals that work in them. As a result, as individual practitioners, we need to consider how we function in teams. The intention of this chapter is to explore issues for you, the individual practitioner, to stimulate your thinking about your own teamworking practices and to give you the opportunity to reflect upon them. You may not agree with all of the inclusions; some may make you smile, some may even irritate or anger you, but hopefully most will make you think. Vygotski (1978) highlighted the importance for us, as teamworkers in learning from each other and those who are only slightly more informed than ourselves. He called this the *zone of proximal development* to encompass the idea that learning is socially and culturally mediated; in simple terms, using those around us to learn. In the same vein, there is of course plenty of academic writing on teamworking for those interested in the finer detail and the research evidence. Whilst some of these are touched on here, this chapter does not set out to be an instructional text based on 'fact' or theory, but rather one to provoke you to think. Direct questions are included from time to time and you are encouraged to explore these from your own perspective. You may even want to put down reading the chapter from time to time until you have done so before proceeding; this might include surveying the opinions of the rest of your team on an issue or question.

SO WHAT IS A TEAM?

Example 5.1

Imagine for a moment the typical locker room pep-talk prior to the World Cup match. The soccer team face the most important match of their professional lives. They are down, but they have the opportunity to fight their way back. Their coach lays it on the line: 'We have a choice here – we can let ourselves get kicked back down into defeat, or we can climb our way back and win. The margin for error is so small. If one of you is half a second or one inch out, it can mean failure for us all. On this team, we must fight for every second and every inch, because that is the difference between winning and losing, living and dying. Each of you has to be willing to die for the other, to sacrifice himself for the team. When you look into the eyes of the guy next to you, you give everything to go the extra inch with him, knowing that he will do the same for you. That's a team.'

The sporting analogy is without doubt the one most often associated with the concept of the team so no apologies are made for starting with one here. This example also gives us a useful agenda for examining the concept of teamworking in health and social care. To me it seems the football coach invites us, as health professionals, to ask ourselves:

- What are the common goals that we are prepared to fight for together to gain the inches in realising them?
- To what extent can we look into the eyes of the fellow professionals in our team and know that there is the sort of interdependence described in the example?
- What is the margin for 'error' in our work that determines our need to work as a team?
- Is the coach's vision of a team anywhere near what we think of in healthcare, or is the concept so different according to context as to be irrelevant?
- Should the concept of the team apply at all in health and social care? Do we work as teams or is it the collective contribution of a number of individuals?
- Are collaborative practice and group working the same or something different; are they complementary or counter-productive to teamwork?

These questions seem to lead us to examine the case for teamworking, our concept of the team and fundamentally, the ways in which we are expected to know how to behave and to work within teams. Finally, they also encourage us to be mindful of the organisational contexts in which health and social care teams operate. As you read the chapter, the questions that should be revisited throughout are: 'What are the common goals, the interdependence and the margin of error that we are prepared to work with each other for?'

Is there a case for teamwork and multi-professional teamworking?

Most health professionals consider the existence of the multi-disciplinary team to be a matter of fact. While there is a widespread view that teamworking and some sort of inter-professional collaboration is a good thing, in the current climate of evidence-based practice there seems to be little to support this.

Zwarenstein et al. (1997) commenting on collaboration, specifically between doctors and nurses, recognised a lack of observable evidence for this improving teamworking. The authors concluded that process indicators, such as inter-disciplinary communication and staff satisfaction are the most significant measures of impact on health and social care. Teram (1997) also cautions us in a similar way, this time to question the unconditional acceptance of the *progressive institutionalisation* of inter-professional teams when they work together for long periods of time. While this may be a very good way of co-ordinating professional working practices, there is the potential conflict that the service user becomes a mere *recipient of care* rather than *a partner in care* as advocated in such edicts as the Health Act 1999. In this way health and social care teams develop a controlling function and *disempower* rather than *empower* service users.

Reflective questions:

- *Who benefits from your team?*
- *Can you identify what these benefits are?*

External drivers and the demand for teamworking

In the present health and social care agenda, a professional or government document cannot be read without failing to come across references to the allied health professions' (AHPs') requirement to work as part of a team. These references are sometimes direct but more often implied through the use of words and concepts such as collaborative practice, working together, partnerships, joined up working, pooling and sharing resources, as well as statements recognising professional boundaries and demonstrating respect for others. All of these paint a united and integrated whole that is perceived as modern health and social care. Consider, for example, the benchmarking statements developed by the AHPs to meet the Quality Assurance Agency (QAA) requirements. These statements have a two-fold purpose and are useful not only for higher education institutions in guiding the development of their curricula and re-validation/ approval of their programmes but also for practitioners by providing the benchmarks for qualifying.

A casual key word search of the physiotherapy statements using terms such as 'team', 'teamwork', 'leader' and 'leadership' highlighted references to physiotherapy's need for teamworking and leadership skills associated with personal and professional development. Also noted was the need for all practitioners to understand both individual and teamworking practice sufficiently to be able to work in both contexts (QAA 2003). There was also a plethora of associated terms that imply teamworking of some sort, for example, 'working with others, negotiation, conciliation, and development of partnerships . . . participate effectively in inter-professional approaches to healthcare delivery' (QAA 2003).

In a similar way an examination of the occupational therapy benchmarking statements reveals much of the same, for example:

- 'Participate effectively in inter-professional and multi-agency approaches to health and social care where appropriate . . .

- Assist other healthcare professionals, support staff and patients/clients/carers in maximising health outcomes . . .
- Recognise the place and contribution of his/her assessment within the total healthcare profile/package through effective communication with other members of the health and social care team . . .
- Build and sustain professional relationships as both an independent practitioner and collaboratively as a member of a team' (QAA 2003).

Interestingly, although there appeared to be no real consistency in the use of the words 'teamworking', 'leadership' or 'leader' in the various professions' benchmarking statements, there was a common thread in the use of the term 'team'. Could this be significant? Is it a case of one assuming that an understanding of the term 'team' infers understanding of and an ability to engage in teamworking and if so, is this correct? A personal view is that it is not, and that this can be the very reason why successful teamworking is so often a matter of chance.

PREPARING FOR TEAMWORK

Professionals leaving higher education should have knowledge and understanding and the necessary skills to participate in a range of teamworking practices and skills in a variety of contexts. This should be valued in the same way as recognition of the ability to carry out individual interventions that are based upon detailed study and practice of them. For example, if we look at any of the benchmarking statements from any of the professions they will all contain the process of assessment of need, planning of intervention, application and evaluation. As such, should not the concept of the team readily reveal the same constructs that have to be understood and practised? Indeed, there should be the same transparency in the learning of all things to do with developing knowledge and skills of teamworking as there is, for example, in the learning of anatomy or a clinical procedure (see Figure 5.1). In the same way teamworking transparency should be seen in clinical practice. If not, where then does the student learn this? Will only those students who happen across a placement

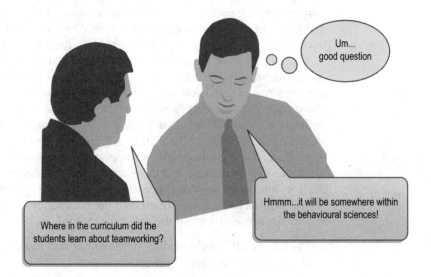

Figure 5.1
A senior academic meeting. Consider: where did you learn about teamworking? Was it explicit or implicit?

where it does work well and is clearly evident develop these skills? Should we tolerate this level of opportunistic learning?

Reflective question:

Consider now whether or not you personally have a good knowledge of teamworking and where this came from, and whether the practice teams you belong to demonstrate this sufficiently clearly.

Gathering pace over the last few years has been the drive for health and social care professions to learn inter-professionally at undergraduate/pre-registration level. Several instances exist; the most ambitious and well known is perhaps the New Generation Project at Southampton and Portsmouth Universities (see also Chapter 4), but there are several others and many instances of small scale ventures.

However, the advent of inter-professional education (IPE) is inconclusive and fraught with difficulties from pedagogical, political and practical perspectives, making it something that is highly variable in design and not yet universally accepted as the way forward. What does seem evident is that the inter-professional learning is increasingly being accepted and included in the strategic plans of higher education institutions, and that IPE is closely associated with the development of increased or improved teamworking amongst health and social care practitioners.

Developing teamworking knowledge and practice as a lifelong learning activity

Teamworking has always been a topic of interest in health and social care arenas. Recent developments, particularly those concerning continuous professional development (CPD) link teamworking with lifelong learning. This is rarely about maintaining the status quo, but about change, and sends out a message of constant evolution of the professions into a cohesive and seamless workforce, namely, a team.

> *Lifelong learning will provide NHS staff with the opportunity to continuously update their skills and knowledge to offer the most modern, effective and high quality care to patients. For example, lifelong learning will allow NHS staff to identify training needs across professions to aid clinical teamworking.*

DoH (1998)

The Health Professions Council (HPC) states that one of its main principles is, 'working collaboratively – the HPC will enable best practice in any one profession to be accessed by all. It will deliver an efficient and unified service as well as focusing on individual issues which are significantly different between professions' (HPC 2003). The list of drivers goes on and on and many examples could be included. Given that there is an overwhelming message to work more collaboratively, to be seen and understood as part of a total healthcare team and to have the skills necessary to operate as a team, do we understand sufficiently what a team is?

SO WHAT IS THIS CONCEPT OF THE TEAM?

Adair (1987) says that the assumption that precise knowledge requires precise definition is wrong; we live with concepts such as energy and light which are not capable of being reduced to simple definition. The same can be said for the concept of the team. We can only begin to make sense of our concepts when they have a specific association of context. Whilst it might be true that a concept by its very nature is an understanding gained by inference and discussed in a generalised way that is context free, the important issue here is that it is for each individual, and in relation to this chapter each team, to make sense for themselves of the concept within their own context.

Child (1984, p. 109) said that, 'The activities of people within an organisation can be grouped to together according to a number of different principles. A functional grouping comprises of people employing a similar expertise. A grouping by process recognises commonalities in plant and technology employed. A product grouping brings together people who are contributing to a common product or service. Other bases for organisationally grouping activities together are their sharing of a similar time horizon or their location on the same physical site.'

In this we can readily identify all the variables that exist in the health and social care setting that adds to any confusion that might exist in the understanding of teamwork.

Some years ago a number of health and social care professionals were surveyed to explore the identity of the teams they felt they were part of (PK Wilby, unpublished work, 1997). The findings suggested that participants defined team memberships with the following common categories:

- By discipline, e.g. the 'medical and nursing team', the 'physiotherapy team', the 'multi-disciplinary team'.
- By geography, e.g. the 'all-Wales speech managers' team'.
- By diagnosis, e.g. 'diabetic teams,' 'cystic fibrosis teams.'
- By function, e.g. the 'facial surgery team,' 'cranio-facial implant team.'

Reflective question:

Can you give a name to the team(s) you belong to, and can it be categorised in a similar way?

The conclusion to be drawn from this is that both teams and the organisations that surround them have to be examined within a specific context, rather than the single professional perspective or a generic account of teamworking. By gaining an insight from different contexts and experiences we can use these to develop a model of teamworking that specifically meets the needs of the organisation and/or task.

Teams and organisations

Paulus (1980) suggested that service organisations are systems made up and developed by people to satisfy human needs. Present health and social services are all complex structures with equally complex functioning. By virtue of their size they can also be very bureaucratic. From both an historical and philosophical view they both conform to well-established hierarchical structures, but this can seem compounded in the health sector due to perceptions of dominance by the medical profession, and perhaps the media headlines about the 'top heavy' management seemingly employed in health. Although a hierarchy also exists in Social Services, the culture at first sight can appear to be flatter and more humanistic due its social rather than medical origins. However the legislative constraints, compartmentalised remit of local government and inflexible management styles can be preclusive for workers in this sector.

'Tall' organisations, containing many hierarchical levels usually have a narrow band of control. This narrow band exists to ensure that each hierarchy only governs a relevant section within the total organisational structure. Health and social care have historically adopted such a model and that has effectively reduced patient/user care into subsections; it is therefore not hard to imagine how difficulties in communication and collaboration between these divisions lead to the loss of service user need as their central focus. Organisations as systems developed by people to meet people's needs would then appear to be in danger of failing to meet the very needs they were designed for. Teram (1997) suggests that teams can be culpable in functioning as a form of social control. As such, professional and organisational cultures should be mindful of the danger of damaging the autonomy of the individual, especially the service user, in their concern over accountability which can lead to an understandable desire for power. As mentioned earlier, this could be seen to be in direct contradiction to the edicts of recent government papers that exhort greater user involvement and patient-centred practices.

The present partnership agenda in health and social care promotes not just teamworking, but collaborative interagency working to such an extent that working practice and culture has to change. As a result structures are becoming flatter and linked. A matrix type model (Figure 5.2) or whole systems method (see Chapter 2) is often used and this requires fluidity in team membership and even role. This may require a more flexible approach to working practice and necessitates clear and effective communication channels.

Strategies such as clinical networks and care pathways are useful to identify best practice in both inter-agency and inter-professional working. Managed clinical networks are linked groups of health professionals and organisations from primary, secondary and tertiary care that work in a co-ordinated manner, unconstrained by existing professional and health board boundaries, to ensure equitable provision of high-quality, clinically effective services (NHS Lothian 2003). Integrated care pathways (ICPs), on the other hand, can be considered as multidisciplinary plans of care that are evidence-based, incorporating national and local guidelines. These form the single clinical record of care for all health professionals involved in the care and treatment of patients/service users (NHS Scotland 2003). In this way the ICP can provide an outline for intervention and can shape how we deliver services in teams. However, ICPs are not cast in stone so should be used only as a guideline to ensure that the most appropriate care is provided (NHS Scotland 2003). This suggests that teams have the flexibility to provide services that meet local needs and professional reasoning can be used in each unique situation.

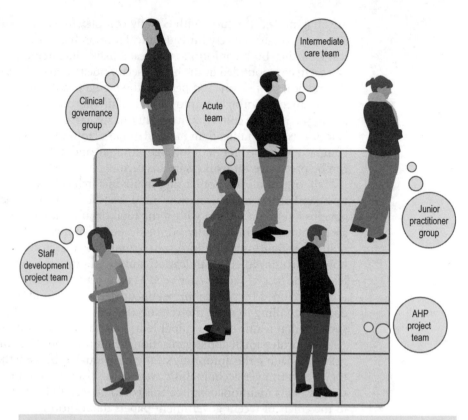

Figure 5.2 In the matrix organisation expertise is professional or skill-based rather than held in personal power or position. The culture in these organisations is one of a team and encourages the development of the group. The culture is flexible and individuals belong to different groups at different times to meet organisational objectives and service user needs. The success of matrix structures is dependent on mutual respect and support in team members. The structure is often compared to a net or web.

Reflective questions:

- *What sort of organisation does your team exist in?*
- *How does the way your team operates reflect the culture of the organisation; is it hierarchically driven or flat?*
- *In what ways does this influence the way your team functions?*
- *What is the basic human need that your team exists to serve and to what extent is the patient/user central to this and in partnership with the team?*
- *If you have a visible user involvement where the user is a partner in your team, how has this changed the team remit, structure and functions?*

Constructing teams

Have you ever thought how you came to be part of your team? Of course this will depend very much on what name you give the team(s) you belong to. If it is the

Table 5.1	Use the following grid to work out how you and your team function				
	What is the team member's profession?	What knowledge base is needed?	What skills are needed?	What is their personality type? (according to Belbin)	What is their actual role in the team?

Modified from Belbin web page: Online. Available: http://www.belbin.com/belbin-team-roles.htm and Belbin M 1981 *Management teams – why they succeed or fail?* Butterworth Heinemann, Oxford.

podiatric or the physiotherapy team then it will probably be by virtue of the qualifications you hold. But what about the alcohol or drug dependency team, the stroke team or the care of the elderly team . . . how was this team 'picked'?

Belbin (1981) described various personalities that co-exist in any group or team, all necessary for contributing to a particularly required role or behaviour. These ranged for example, from the 'company-worker' to the 'team-worker'. The former is described as being conservative, dutiful and predictable, a good organiser, with lots of practical common sense, hard working and self-disciplined. They can also lack flexibility and be unresponsive to unproven ideas at times. The latter is described as a person who is socially orientated, rather mild, and sensitive. They have an ability to respond to people and situations and to promote team spirit. However, they can be indecisive at moments of crisis. There are several other 'types' that Belbin describes as having a role within the team. Copy the grid in Table 5.1 and then list the members of your team, completing the questions for each of them . . . does the team look well balanced in terms of what each is providing? Is equal attention paid to the personalities that make up the team as well as the knowledge and skills they bring to it? You may wish to carry out the Belbin questionnaire with your colleagues before doing this, or you may just ascribe a personality according to your best understanding of them. The Belbin inventory can be found at http://www.belbin.com/belbin-team-roles.htm

Unique personalities can cause conflicts within teams. Strategies to understand our own behaviour and to deal with difficult people can be useful and are an important aspect of teamworking. It is worth considering how you can use techniques such as negotiation skills to enable effective service delivery. Where there are apparently insurmountable barriers in communication and working patterns, changes in our own behaviour can often overcome these and thus achieve both positive working relationships and quality outcomes.

A PERSON-CENTRED APPROACH TO HEALTH AND SOCIAL CARE

A person-centred approach encourages a view of relationships from each participant's standpoint. A person-centred philosophy encompasses the individual as a member of the team as well as someone who exists outside of the team and subsumes both positions as one. As a result, this approach takes more account of what might commonly be seen as peripheral factors.

The more often heard term of client- or patient-centredness (and in education student-centredness) has a narrower focus. It deals with the individual solely as a recipient of care. From the team perspective it could be said that its equivalent, the multi-disciplinary team approach is similarly narrow, seeing team members only in terms of their discipline-specific contribution. West (1994) identifies this as when a team only operates in respect of the tasks it is expected to perform, i.e. 'task reflexivity', at the expense of seeing the people in the team, i.e. 'social reflexivity'. Too much of the former results in ultimately poor mental health and the risk of 'burn-out'; too much of the latter can mean lack of productivity and mental lethargy. Adopting a person-centred approach not only ensures that the client or patient is regarded as more than the sum of his/her pathology (what is often rhetorically described as a holistic approach), but it also ensures the same for the members of the team. Teams then, are developed and operated according not only to the professional knowledge and skills required but also the human requirements that are needed for what is, fundamentally, a socially functioning group. This, in part, encapsulates the sort of attributes that Belbin and his contemporaries describe, but also those simple human qualities of caring and sharing that are required and that determine the 'social reflexivity' of the team.

Reflective exercises:

- Consider your area of work and identify what the needs of the patient/client/user are and those of the team if they are to function effectively through recognising the person aspects of the team.
- 'Pick' your team for this area of work and see if it is the same as already exists . . . even if it means you have a changed role or even no role at all . . . in an evidenced-based culture we have to consider this possibility before others do it for us!

CONCLUSION

Have you identified what that common goal is that is shared by your team, the inches that are needed to achieve them? How comfortable are you about looking into the eye of your fellow team-worker and knowing they are vital to your success and the team's? If you are not, what are you going to do about it? What ever it is, good luck!

REFERENCES

Adair J 1987 *Effective teambuilding: how to make a winning team.* Pan, London.
Belbin M 1981 *Management teams – why they succeed or fail?* Butterworth Heinemann, Oxford.
Child J 1984 *Organisations: A guide to problems and practice.* Harper Row, London.
Department of Health 1998 *A first class service: quality in the new NHS.* Department of Health, London.
Department of Health 2001 *Shifting the balance of power in the NHS: securing delivery.* Department of Health, London.
Department of Health 2002 *Shifting the balance of power in the NHS: the next steps.* Department of Health, London.
Health Act 1999 HMSO, London.
Health Professions Council 2003
    Online. Available:
    http://www.hpc-uk.org/about_us/aims_vision.htm.
    11 September 2003.

NHS Lothian 2003 *Managed clinical networks*. NHS Lothian.
Online. Available:
http://www.nhslothian.scot.nhs.uk/publications/annual_reports/public_health/2002/18/
1 February 2003.
NHS Scotland 2003 *Integrated care pathways*. NHS Scotland.
Online. Available:
http://www.show.scot.nhs.uk/nhsfv/clineff/icp/ICPs.htm.
1 February 2003.
Paulus NL 1980 *The organisation in its environment*. Polytech Publishers, Stockport.
Quality Assurance Agency (QAA) 2003 *Subject benchmark statements*.
Online. Available:
http://www.qaa.ac.uk.
12 June 2003.
Teram E 1997 Interdisciplinary teams and the control of clients: a sociotechnical perspective.
Human Relations 44(4): 343–356.
Vygotski LS 1978 *The mind in society: the development of higher psychological processes*. Harvard
Press, Cambridge.
West MA 1994 *Effective teamwork*. The British Psychological Society, London.
Zwarenstein M, Bryant W, Baillie R, Sibthorpe B 1997 Interventions to change collaboration
between nurses and doctors. *The Cochrane Library Issues* 2: 1–11.

RECOMMENDED READING

Handy C 1993 *Understanding organisations*, 4th edn. Penguin, London.
* A great book for understanding how organisations work.
Lilley R 2003 *Dealing with difficult people*. Kogan Page, London.
* Fantastic little book that gives tips on working with difficult people.
West MA 2003 *Effective teamwork: practical lessons from organisational research*. Blackwell,
Oxford.
* Another cracker from this excellent writer.
West MA, Markiewicz L 2003 *Building team-based working: a practical guide to organisational
transformation*. Blackwell, London.
* Thoughtful and practical ideas on effective teamworking.

6 Continuing professional development

Lyn Westcott

LEARNING OUTCOMES

- Clarify concept of CPD and why it is important for allied health professionals.
- Delineate statutory elements of CPD.
- Outline some structures and models used to facilitate CPD in the workplace (including supervision, mentoring and appraisal).
- Identify and explore a range of tools to enhance your professional development.
- Examine how to develop a professional profile that fits your own needs and compile a CPD file.
- Clarify the academic structure of post-qualification development.

INTRODUCTION

Being a practising member of an allied health profession (AHP) brings different responsibilities and expectations than other types of non-professional employment. Practitioners are expected to move alongside developments in their field and shape these changes using their expertise. This is enabled by participation in 'continuing professional development' (CPD).

This chapter aims to describe and discuss CPD from both a theoretical and practical viewpoint. This will help you develop an understanding of what CPD is and why it is relevant to each AHP practitioner, the users of their services and their employers. It will also assist in identifying how a range of measures can help to facilitate the CPD process at an organisational, departmental and individual practitioner level.

WHAT IS CPD AND WHY IS IT IMPORTANT?

Professional practice is more than holding down a job where clearly defined skills are learnt and used by employees, who may not feel responsibility to change them over time. Practitioners are expected to move actively together with perpetual ongoing developments in their field, using these changes to shape and evolve their expertise. This not only provides practitioners with a never-ending process of professional and personal growth but also benefits service users and providers with staff able to deliver dynamic and topical patterns of practice in an ever changing and developing world. Remember that a person qualifying within an AHP could have over 40 years of practice before they retire. It is totally unrealistic and naive to think that everything they will need to know over this time will be covered in their basic pre-registration study. Times change and knowledge develops; alongside this the health and social care sectors evolve with differing expectations placed upon their workers. The necessary ongoing

Figure 6.1
CPD –
principles for
practitioners
and
environmental
influences.
Modified from
CSP (2002).

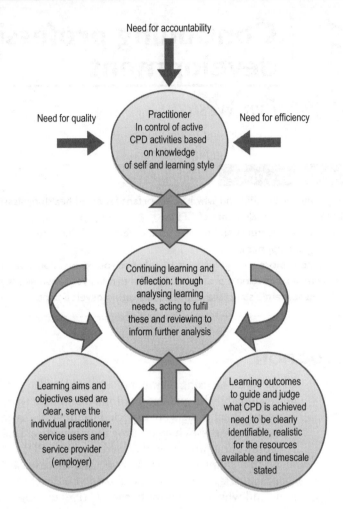

personal process of change, required to keep up with the new demands on practitioners is formalised and recognised under the umbrella term of 'continuing professional development' (CPD).This is an important part of the wider government-driven agenda of 'lifelong learning', a broad concept that encapsulates necessary ongoing progression in knowledge, thinking and skills development for all levels of health and social care workers (including support staff). These concepts fit well with the sense of professional responsibility that are reasonably expected of an AHP and therefore required at a professional and regulatory level. The Code of Ethics and Professional Conduct for Occupational Therapists (COT 2000, Section 5) for example, identifies active CPD as a condition of practice, whilst the HPC is also introducing regulation to this end (HPC 2003a). This is reflected in the HPC Standards of Conduct, Performance and Ethics (2003) which states that registrants must keep their 'professional knowledge and skills up to date' (Section 5). Whilst recognised as vital at a higher level, CPD is seen as something that is the responsibility of the individual professional. It is the practitioner who is expected to be an active instigator and participant in this process. Figure 6.1 illustrates some fundamental elements of CPD in this respect, showing the practitioner within a professional practice context that reflects the current demands of ongoing change. As a member of an AHP, each individual practitioner needs to demonstrate clearly their continuous updating of skills and perpetual development of professionalism at work.

Statutory elements of CPD

Demonstration of active learning to keep up to date with professional knowledge and skills is a requirement of the Health Professions Council (HPC). Evidence supporting an individual's CPD can be monitored at any time by the HPC from 2006, they will have the power to remove a practitioner from the UK register for their profession. The process of CPD is reflective of quality priorities identified by UK Government and Department of Health (DoH) in the form of Clinical Governance for Health, Best Value in Local Government (see also Chapters 1 and 7) and moves such as the Generic Post Graduate Learning Framework, a strategy that is emergent at the time of writing this chapter (see http://www.doh.gov.uk).

The HPC derived from the Health Professions Act (1999) and replaced the Council for Professions Supplementary to Medicine in April 2002, under the Health Professions Council Order (Great Britain 2002). It was established with a wider remit than the body it supplanted, based on the need to demonstrate clearly full professional status for each profession and their members enrolled on HPC registers. This includes active self-regulation and consistency in terms of quality and professionally fit practitioners. At the time the HPC was formed this applied to 12 health professions including chiropodists and podiatrists, occupational therapists, radiographers, physiotherapists and speech and language therapists. The number of professions included is planned to increase over time. The 'Protection of Title' aspect of the HPC registers means that only those on HPC registers can practise with that job title in the UK.

One of the major remits for the new HPC is to set up and monitor a system for CPD that is linked to this duty to register those considered fit to practise. The passage to initial registration is through completion of an approved curriculum, whilst the ability to remain on the register (and practise), means registrants must prove that they meet the minimum CPD requirements set by the HPC. This system therefore formalises what responsible registrants have been doing for years, i.e. fulfilling their duty to maintain their skills in an up to date way. The process of development however no longer relies on the good will of individuals or their employers as it has in the past. There is a new policing element being introduced that can de-register those who cannot prove they are CPD active. This system cannot be detailed in this chapter (as it is still emergent at the time of writing); the HPC have announced their intention probably to introduce re-registration requirements in 2006 (HPC 2003b). What can be safely assumed however is that national minimal standards for CPD will apply and this will require active commitment from registrants, not just a monitoring of hours that might count as CPD time (HPC 2003b). HPC will select a proportion of registrants annually to examine CPD activity (HPC 2004). The CPD portfolio can be a useful resource to hold and focus CPD activity and reflection by individual practitioners, providing a clear set of documentary evidence from which practitioners can select relevant information to demonstrate their learning and development in the required format for HPC. This portfolio can also be produced to employers and the HPC as a running record of career development over time (for suggested contents see below). All registrants with the HPC already sign a declaration stating that they keep up to date with professional knowledge and skills when they re-register their status with this body. Any recent requirements for CPD by the HPC will be available via their website (www.hpc-uk.org).

Structures, processes and models used to facilitate CPD in the workplace (including supervision, mentoring and appraisal)

Employing organisations in health and social care have evolved structures to manage their human resources, ensuring that individuals are able to fulfil the expectations of their post and demonstrate a level of competence expected within that role. These are generally formal, often including documentation processes. In tandem with this, professionals have evolved support mechanisms that reflect their professional aspirations for excellence in practice; these have been embedded in some areas for many years, e.g. palliative care and mental health. In other areas they are less common, although they are gaining more recognition as valuable for supporting employees in stressful work environments. You should be involved at least in the former of these two categories in any health or social care AHP position.

Every AHP practitioner, even those in the most senior positions, require regular supervision to ensure they are fulfilling their job description in an optimum way. This is of benefit to the employee and employer, monitoring and supporting the performance, satisfaction and growth of an individual within an organisation. Supervision may vary in its style (see Figure 6.2), depending on need. It should always be a formal and regular process with a written record of aims and objectives set to enable the employee to achieve their potential on a day to day basis within that post. The styles most reflective of current CPD practice are 'personal growth' and 'educational'. These can easily be recorded in reflective content, achievement synopsis and development plan of a CPD portfolio (see below). The supervision process enables and ensures fitness for purpose in the work role so that employees fulfil their duty to service users.

In addition to supervision and supplementary to its function as a monitoring process, some employees may also be offered mentoring by a more experienced colleague/professional. This is a less formalised mechanism for reflection and support separate from the management agenda that governs supervision. For this reason it is not wise to accept supervision and mentoring from the same person, as both parties may be trapped in an awkward position of potential role conflict. Mentorship should be a place for exploration and reflection on a range of issues; this is different from working towards and monitoring targets of achievement. Mentorship may be individual or take the form of support groups, a format familiar to mental health settings for example. Sometimes mentorship may be appropriately provided by a colleague from another discipline, for example within a specialist practice team having only one person from a particular AHP.

As part of the conditions of public sector employment, you should expect at least an annual formal appraisal of your performance with your nominated manager. This is linked to local clinical governance procedures (in health), and often called an interim performance review (IPR), the chosen term for this chapter. This is a formal, documented, two way interview that details achievements in the previous year and sets targets for the year ahead. This can be of

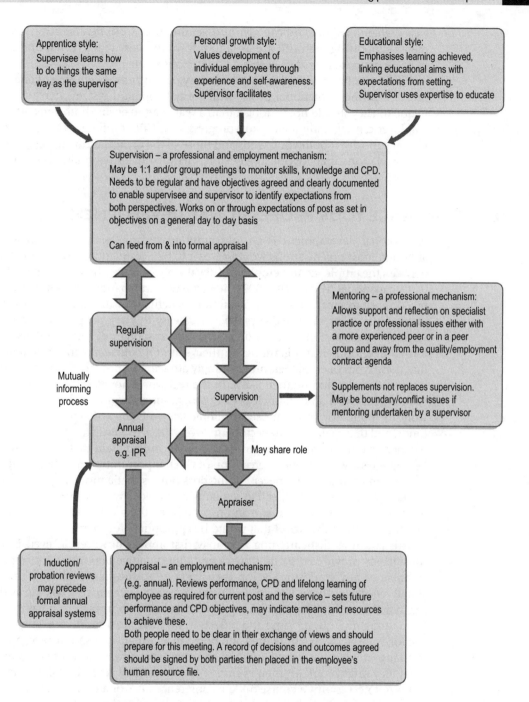

Figure 6.2 Overview of supervision and appraisal processes.

benefit to both employer and employee by acknowledging and valuing the contribution of the post holder. It clarifies what you expect of your work and what is expected of you in the year ahead. It also documents development needs and identifies further training that should be completed or other means to address these. It is important to approach these sessions thoughtfully and be well prepared so that you can give and get the most from this occasion. Documents supporting each IPR are used to inform the next year's review and need to be an accurate record of events and decisions made.

Sometimes (such as during a probationary period at the beginning of employment or during a rotational post), these formal appraisal systems may be more frequent. They should not be longer than a year apart to ensure both you and your employer can regularly review and progress your CPD profile in a collaborative way, ensuring that both your needs and those of the organisation are being met.

The relationship between supervision, mentorship and appraisal is shown in Figure 6.2.

TOOLS TO ENHANCE YOUR PROFESSIONAL DEVELOPMENT

Professional development is an inherently active process by each individual, although most organisations would agree it to be a joint approach at some level between the employer and employee (Royal College of Psychiatrists and College of Occupational Therapists 2002). It involves participation and effort by the practitioner to create and gain maximum benefit from the opportunities that inevitably present in everyday practice. It is easy to envy people who seem to work for organisations with endless time and resources devoted to delivering formal development programmes to their staff. Of course, it cannot be denied that these types of employers are seemingly attractive, especially for practitioners interested in developing their skills. In the real world however it might be hard to find posts with abundant clear CPD programmes as most AHP practitioners work for public or voluntary sector employers with limited staff development funds, and those with private sector employers practise within a system that must balance investment costs with profits gained. It could be said that there seems to be a 'grass is always greener' perception of CPD opportunities in different organisations and few meet the never-ending possibilities that a motivated individual would have on their wish list. Do remember that like any ongoing process, CPD is by its very nature without end and no one (even the most fortunate) is able to do all the CPD in the world that would be appropriate for them!

This is not as disheartening as it may first appear however, as even in the most leanly provided organisation, there can be positive opportunities for practitioners of any grade to develop their CPD opportunities, skills and professional reflection. This is because CPD cannot be a passive process; as long as you can practise and reflect you can achieve sound CPD. Someone can gain more from thoughtful questioning and reflection on their most mundane daily practice for example, than sitting tired and bored in an expensive training programme thinking of what happened last night in their favourite soap on television or what they might cook for their evening meal when they get home! CPD can be, but is not necessarily, a course on X, a conference on Y or a training symposium from an international expert open only to selected individuals that does not include yourself. CPD is available to everyone in several different ways; the real problem is that sometimes people fail to identify and use what could be an ideal opportunity for personal and professional growth and development. The essence of the CPD process therefore is to seek out and recognise the opportunities that are presented, create more where you can, and be active in your reflection and development processes.

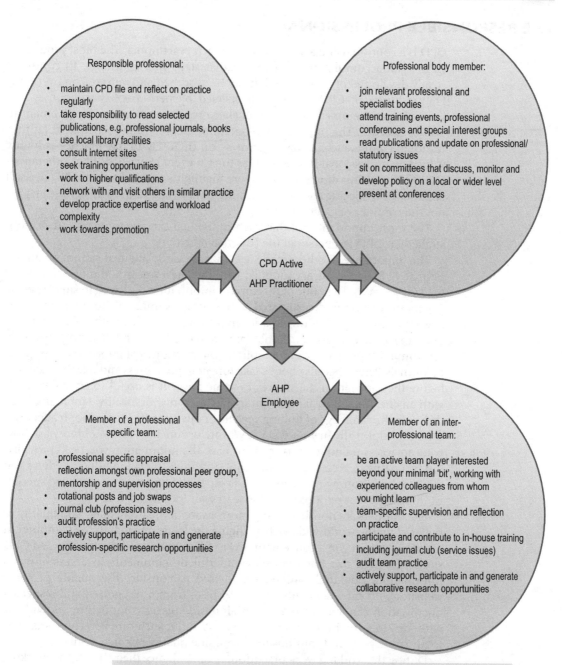

Figure 6.3 Example opportunities for CPD by a development aware practitioner.

Demonstrating active and ongoing CPD say in a personal file (see section below), not only proves to yourself that you are continuing to develop over time, but also helps to show your employer and professional organisations like the Health Professions Council (HPC), that you value and are active in your personal and professional growth. Some of the ways CPD can be undertaken are illustrated in Figure 6.3.

THE RESPONSIBLE PROFESSIONAL

CPD is a continual and active process by each practitioner. The most productive CPD is an accumulation of small, regular steps that contribute to continual steady development in practice that can be absorbed and reflected on over time. Frantic bursts of CPD activity interspersed by periods of inaction may feel impacting at the time but are less likely to result in enduring improvement in skill or practice. The importance of enabling people to demonstrate their professional competence in ways that draw on their day to day practice is highly valued by professional bodies such as the Chartered Society of Physiotherapists (CSP) (2002). This discussion therefore highlights possibilities for CPD beyond attendance at specific courses or training days which (although significant) are not the confines of CPD activity.

The most important tool that each individual can use to focus and demonstrate their CPD is a personal file (discussed below).

The importance of other small steps that are easily attained cannot be underestimated. Practitioners are supplied with the latest research and debate in their field via journals. The value of this topical information packaged in small specific papers cannot be underestimated, but is only helpful to those who read it! Beware of the trap of allowing a journal to lie unopened with good intention until the next one arrives. Books are well respected and helpful (especially for complex topics), but cannot replicate the recentness of information supplied in journals. This is because books take longer to go to press and may be outdated before they appear on the shelves in some areas. It is useful to equate yourself with any health and social care library facilities in your locality. Librarians often thrive on the challenge of finding specific or obscure information for readers and can be a helpful ally in your CPD. If you are unsure how to use a library ask how you can access training – it is tragic to have the information you need provided but be unable to access it. Welcome opportunities to read in libraries where you may not have borrowing rights – this is especially important if you need specialist information or resources and those in your locality are limited.

Practitioners are now becoming more aware of the immediacy and quality of material on the world-wide-web, bringing the latest research to the computer in the office or home in a convenient way to fill snatches of time or dedicated CPD slots. Although this has marked wonderful developments in accessibility to information, potential 'surfers' are advised to consider the quality of some websites with care. Remember that a website from a recognised and respected organisation can appear in a search alongside pieces compiled by individuals with axes to grind in their garden sheds! Without such care you could inadvertently value poor and spurious text alongside quality research evidence.

During the working week practitioners can enhance their CPD by networking and visiting colleagues with similar work-loads. Negotiating with more senior staff to work jointly with more difficult or specialist case-work may help develop skills towards promotion or discretionary points within a given pay scale.

The professional body member

All AHP staff are advised to join their professional body who is able to support and contribute to its members' CPD. Specialist practitioners may choose to join additional uni- or multi-professional organisations with this end in mind. Members are made aware of opportunities for research and development organised by each professional body, many offering training events, conferences to disseminate innovative practice and changes in service provision. Some professional bodies also hold specialist interest groups for practitioners and students within particular working areas to meet and share information – these may suit some people's CPD needs more than generalist professional events. The professional bodies for AHPs have worked hard to meet the need for quality self-regulation inferred upon them by the Health Professions Council Order (Great Britain 2002) and maintain their tradition for supporting their members' CPD through issuing profession-specific publications and guidelines that shape and report on practice.

As a member of a professional body, it is easy to forget that your role need not be confined to being at the receiving end of the work done on your behalf. The organisations are generally fairly small compared to the number of registered practitioners they serve. The quality of their work depends on active support from members that forward action in a range of areas; this occurs on local as well as national level throughout the UK. You can gain CPD within your profession by getting involved for example in the running of committees to discuss, monitor and develop policy on a local or wider level. By becoming involved even at a local level you are more likely to influence the type of CPD opportunities organised in your area. It may even inspire you to collaborate or develop some CPD for colleagues yourself! Active involvement in this way is certainly excellent networking at any stage of your career.

The member of a profession-specific team

Irrespective of their setting, most AHP practitioners either work within or can access contact with a profession-specific team. This contact is especially important to maintain profession-specific CPD as isolation from your own peers can lead to loss of morale and direction, even for confident autonomous practitioners. All practitioners should work within some mechanism that accesses regular supervision and appraisal of their professional skills. Newer practitioners should expect both of these roles to be undertaken by more senior staff from their discipline and may have an additional mentor to talk through issues specific to their particular service. Senior staff may need to be more inventive to obtain supervision. The essence of these procedures for CPD is that they allow a practitioner to think through and reflect on their development within the workplace, gaining support and encouragement to fulfil the needs of their post. Appraisal procedures are usually annual events, although may be more frequent for people working rotational posts. They formalise the review of personal attainment and goal setting for future development by recording goals for specific CPD. Appraisal should be a positive process consolidating issues that have formed the basis for supervision throughout the year. They are an ideal opportunity to document agreement for specific CPD measures that have been identified by the individual as important and give a firm benchmark to review progress next time.

Some organisations have rotational posts especially for newer practitioners that enable CPD to be gained through experiencing different aspects of the service for that profession in the locality. These are ideal for newer practitioners who want to consolidate a range of skills or are uncertain of where to specialise.

Rotational posts typically move people on at 6-monthly intervals, although this may be longer periods for posts with more seniority or speciality. For senior practitioners individually negotiated rotation or job swapping arrangements over fixed timescales can develop practitioners across a service at a higher level, offering opportunities for hands-on transferability of skills and reflection.

Many AHPs have regular profession-specific meetings across a locality that can offer contact for peers from more isolated posts. These forums can be exploited to include CPD issues such as journal clubs to discuss and critique papers of mutual interest. They also provide networking opportunities to share and disseminate local practice. Working within a particular service or locality offers opportunities for practitioners to gather and evaluate the evidence gathered within their practice. This information is important as it is specifically valid to the service users in that place. Profession-specific teams may use formalised tools such as audit, to track evidence and procedure on certain issues. It is also feasible for groups to think through more formalised research opportunities within their area, supporting and working collaboratively within their professional group.

The member of an inter-professional team

Many AHP practitioners may find themselves working as the only representative of their profession or one of a small peer team within a larger mixed professional group. Although this means individuals may have to make greater effort to contact their own professional peers for CPD, they have the benefits of learning from colleagues with different skills about a specialist area of practice. To optimise on the opportunities in these posts it is important to be an active team player with an interest wider than your minimal 'bit'. Some specialist areas such as mental health, may involve some generic working and whilst it is important to maintain your professional autonomy and focus, much can be gained in CPD terms from joint working across disciplines, especially with more experienced practitioners. Some teams have inter-disciplinary supervision on practice issues, which can complement and broaden thinking on challenging areas. This can contribute important material for reflection in a CPD file. Many teams have in-house training events that give useful opportunities to develop specialist skills. You may decide to contribute to the CPD of others by facilitating an event from your own professional perspective. Inter-professional teams can instigate service- rather than profession-specific audit, providing a unique CPD opportunity into that particular service. As with profession-specific initiatives, the inter-disciplinary forum enables AHP workers to actively support, participate in and generate collaborative research opportunities with a service- rather than discipline-specific agenda.

Developing a professional profile that fits your own needs and compiling a CPD file

Your personal profile of competency and professionalism as a practitioner will continue to develop as your expertise grows. This is fed by your accumulating knowledge, experiences and skill development gained at college then during each post and educational opportunity you take up. This should not however be an ad hoc process and needs to be thought through carefully to reflect both the opportunities afforded to you and your continuous appraisal of your own development needs over time. The action elements of this are guided by devising and formulating learning aims, objectives and an action plan for yourself that is subject to regular reflection, action and review (see Figure 6.1). You may decide to use your mentoring or supervision processes to inform this but essentially your professional profile is personal to you.

A professional development portfolio in the form of a file is an accepted way to document your professional profile. It provides a focused means to centralise, hold and track your CPD as your career unfolds. CPD files are fluid, dynamic resources that will need regular revision as your own CPD needs develop and grow. Your portfolio 1 year after qualifying should become very different in its content and focus 10 years later. Although detailed reflection on incidents in your first post may usefully inform your junior practice years, you will find that those details become less relevant when your skills and reflections move onto more specialised or complex areas of practice. This editing process ensures your file is current in its focus and relevant to your present development needs. It also ensures that the content is kept at a manageable size, retaining its usefulness and readability, drawing on selected highlights rather than the minutiae of all the component parts of your professional experience!

You may decide that there are parts of your portfolio that are not appropriate to share, such as your personal reflections on particular experiences in practice. If you decide to use your portfolio to support a job application or inform a supervision or educational session, it is acceptable to remove such material for that occasion.

There are no hard and fast rules governing the precise contents of a portfolio although factual and reflective elements should be included. The content does need to be organised however with logical and meaningful sequencing. Some suggestions on content are included in Figure 6.4.

These guidelines can be adapted to any stage in your career from student to senior practitioner. Portfolios can help to synthesise experiences when preparing for formal review of your post or enabling you to prepare for major change such as seeking a new post or promotion. They can also provide evidence of your CPD on demand such as by the HPC. Although a portfolio centres on the individual practitioner, it also provides evidence of that practitioner's role in relation to the service users they work with and employer they serve. These interests need some kind of synergy if the practitioner is to work effectively.

OUTLINE OF THE ACADEMIC STRUCTURE FOR POST-QUALIFICATION DEVELOPMENT

In the UK the pre-registration education of AHPs is held in the higher education and sometimes further education sectors. Higher education includes those institutions within the university system; further education colleges enrol school leavers who are working to enter university or gain vocational qualifications, usually at levels below a degree award.

All of the programmes for AHPs are written by academic teams, informed by guidance from their professional body, the HPC and other quality mechanisms in higher education such as the Quality Assurance Agency (QAA). Programmes are designed so that successful students can satisfy at least the minimum needs of qualified practitioners for their profession and be allowed to register with the HPC. The HPC is developing curriculum guidance that outlines minimum competencies

Figure 6.4
Components of
a CPD portfolio.
Modified from
Fenech (1999).

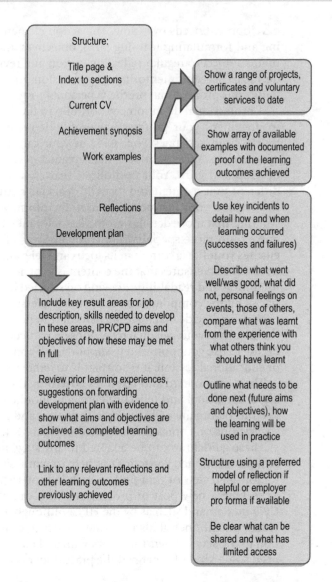

Structure:

Title page &
Index to sections

Current CV

Achievement synopsis

Work examples

Reflections

Development plan

Show a range of projects,
certificates and voluntary
services to date

Show array of available
examples with documented
proof of the learning
outcomes achieved

Use key incidents to
detail how and when
learning occurred
(successes and failures)

Describe what went
well/was good, what did
not, personal feelings on
events, those of others,
compare what was learnt
from the experience with
what others think you
should have learnt

Outline what needs to be
done next (future aims
and objectives), how
the learning will be
used in practice

Structure using a preferred
model of reflection if
helpful or employer
pro forma if available

Be clear what can be
shared and what has
limited access

Include key result areas for job
description, skills needed to develop
in these areas, IPR/CPD aims and
objectives of how these may be met
in full

Review prior learning experiences,
suggestions on forwarding
development plan with evidence to
show what aims and objectives are
achieved as completed learning
outcomes

Link to any relevant reflections and
other learning outcomes
previously achieved

across their governed professions with this in mind (due July 2005 – see www.hpc-uk.org for details). The professional bodies also devise curriculum guidance from their position of expertise and these have governed each AHP curriculum up to the creation of HPC. They will continue to inform the emergent curriculum standards of HPC. Alongside this, universities are generally mindful of the need to involve both HPC and professional body expertise in curriculum formation and approval, reflecting both sets of requirements in their curricula. Radiography programmes for example have generally been devised to satisfy the curriculum guidelines of the Society of Radiographers (2003), and occupational therapy, the standards of the College of Occupational Therapists (2003). How these will be absorbed in educational practice as the HPC continues to develop and define its role will be of interest.

In addition to AHP professional organisations, curricula also reflect the educational philosophy of the particular academic team in the way the programme is delivered. A pre-registration programme may therefore have problem-based learning elements (where students research and discuss work in small groups), or a timetable of only lectures and more formalised learning. Different programmes will offer various opportunities for inter-professional education and learning, often with other AHP students or perhaps nurses, medical students or social workers. Whatever the style of any individual programme, each is regularly approved and monitored and at the time of writing the usual interval has been 5 years. Under the new HPC arrangements of programme approval this may change (see www.hpc-uk.org). Programme approvals recognise the interests and standards of the educational institution, the HPC and respective professional body. This is to ensure that successful finalists from every approved institution can register for practice as fit, able and up to date practitioners, and become part of their professional body.

The levels of minimum academic attainment required by each profession to gain registration with the HPC will vary and some programmes will give academic awards above the minimum required; for example, a physiotherapy or occupational therapy practitioner may earn a pre-registration MSc when the minimum requirement for registration is BSc (Hons). The level of academic award is generally tied to the time spent in study and the level of complexity successfully completed in that learning. This is important when thinking through the transferability of an individual's qualification when coming from or going to practice overseas, different countries have varying acceptability thresholds for qualifications required by their practitioners. This will mean that some nationals will hold levels of qualifications higher than those required within the UK whilst others will not satisfy the minimum requirements. Professional bodies are responsible for scrutinising the acceptability of overseas qualifications in the UK to regulate professional standards. British practitioners often have to adhere to similar processes when seeking to work overseas.

The system of academic levels is not just important for pre-registration students or hopeful HPC registrants from overseas, as qualified practitioners can also study programmes that contribute to or complete the requirements of additional academic qualifications. Higher education institutions may insist on completion of a certain level of award before progressing with higher study at their institution, e.g. a Bachelors degree to enter a Masters programme, or Masters to begin PhD. On the positive side, they often allow attainment gained at different places to be carried forward and topped up with extra study, especially for post-registration students who do not need specific qualifications to register for practice. Institutions count both old and new study elements towards another exit award that can be given under a credit accumulation transfer scheme (CATS) or accredited prior learning (APL). It is therefore important to bear in mind the level and contribution possibilities that can be gained by completing a particular programme if you want to achieve another qualification as part of your CPD. Higher levels of attainment are regarded as solid evidence of career development and are increasingly valued and recognised as currency for AHPs entering higher levels of practice such as Head or Consultant Therapist posts. Table 6.1 shows how levels of award are determined in England and Wales (Scotland and Ireland require 120 additional credits for Bachelors with Honours).

In addition to striving for formal qualifications, active CPD may also be used by individuals to support promotion or aid their defence in disciplinary cases. A thorough record of CPD can be used in the evaluation of an individual's capacity to fulfil their job description, supporting their case during disciplinary

Table 6.1	Minimum academic credits for defined exit awards, England and Wales
Minimum credits required	**Exit award given**
120 credits at Level I	Certificate in Higher Ed.
Plus 120 credits at Level II	Diploma in Higher Ed. (Equivalent to Foundation degree)
Plus 60 credits at Level III	Bachelors (Ordinary)
or 120 credits at Level III	Bachelors with Honours
60 credits Masters level	Postgraduate Certificate
120 credits Masters level	Postgraduate Diploma
180 credits Masters level	Masters degree
	(Doctorate level study PhD)

Notes: One credit normally equates to 10 hours of study, 120 credits being 1200 hours or 1 year of typical full time academic year attendance. Some Masters programmes may not be offered using modules and will not allocate credits in this way, doctorate level study is not credit rated.

hearings or conversely aiding promotion or re-grading under formal mechanism such as those worked through in health under The Agenda for Change (see Chapter 1).

CONCLUSION

This chapter has discussed CPD and its importance to AHP practitioners from a statutory, professional and personal viewpoint. Some means to enhance CPD have been suggested and components of a CPD portfolio outlined. CPD is an emergent area of the upmost importance to each AHP. The structures that validate and guide CPD are evolving at the time of writing this chapter. This chapter can help you understand the need for your own CPD and optimise opportunities as they present. In this climate of development and change, readers are strongly advised to consult their particular professional body and the HPC to ensure they conform with the most current requirements for CPD.

Exercise 1

(a) Complete a 'SWOT' analysis (list of Strengths, Weaknesses, Opportunities and Threats) for the CPD opportunities in your ideal post – consider both what the post offers you and what you can actively contribute to it.

(b) Compare the 'SWOT' for (a) above with a second 'SWOT' for your current post or most recent practice placement and note the points of difference – again consider both what the post/placement offers/offered you and what you actively contribute/d.

(c) How can you make the best of the opportunities in (b) to turn them into strengths? How might you utilise the strengths in this environment to minimise the effect of any weaknesses? How might you deal with the threats to enhance your CPD?

Exercise 2

Examine the figure of CPD opportunities – how many apply to you in your present post or most recent placement? Identify one short-, one medium- and one long-term goal for your own CPD based on these or other suggestions. Devise a plan in your CPD file to work towards these.

Exercise 3

Clarify the HPC requirements for re-registration in your profession. What can be fulfilled by activities that you can instigate yourself (see Exercises 1 and 2)? How can you best document these processes? Are there sections that clearly show these requirements in your CPD file?

Useful websites

Department of Health.
http://doh.gov.uk

Health Professions Council.
http://www.hpc-uk.org

REFERENCES

Chartered Society of Physiotherapists 2002 *Lifelong learning-competence*
Online. Available:
http://.csp.org.uk/lifelonglearning/competance/cpd.cfm
25 June 03.
College of Occupational Therapists 2000 *The code of ethics and professional conduct for occupational therapists*. College of Occupational Therapists, London.
College of Occupational Therapists 2003 *Standards for education: pre-registration education standards*. College of Occupational Therapists, London.
Fenech A 1999 The A–Z of continuing professional development: part three, creating a portfolio. *Occupational Therapy News* November: 12–13.
Great Britain 2002 *The Health Professions Order 2001. (Transitional provisions) order 2002. (Statutory Instrument 1124)*. Stationery Office, London.
Health Professions Act 1999. Stationery Office, London.
Health Professions Council 2004 *Continuing Professional Development – Consultation Paper*
Online. Available:
http://www.hpc-uk.org
3 March 2005.
Health Professions Council 2003a *Standards of conduct, performance and ethics; your duties as a registrant*. Health Professions Council, London.
Health Professions Council 2003b *Registrants – continuing professional development*
Online. Available:
http://www.hpc-uk.org/registrants/cpd.htm
21 Nov 03.
Royal College of Psychiatrists and College of Occupational Therapists 2002 *Mental health and occupation in participation*. Royal College of Psychiatrists and College of Occupational Therapists. London.
Society of Radiographers 2003 *Curriculum framework for radiography*. Deesons, London.

7

Aspects of professionalism – factors influencing allied health practice

Gwilym Wyn Roberts

LEARNING OUTCOMES

■ Discussion of professionalism for AHPs linked to lifelong learning, continuing professional development (CPD) and continued competence to practise.
■ Delineating the purpose of pre-registration education and the way new AHPs are prepared for professional practice.
■ Outlining the role of codes of ethics and professional conduct in guiding professional practice.
■ Consideration of the human potential of AHPs to further develop their specialist skills through role of continuing professional development and research, including how this expertise can influence their choice of careers as managers and/or consultant therapists.
■ Exploring the organisational boundaries within which professional practice occurs, identifying some important drivers, changes, opportunities and challenges for AHPs in health and social care.

INTRODUCTION

This chapter will examine the nature of professionalism and the way in which allied health professionals (AHPs) need to adapt, develop and synthesise their knowledge, experience and skills. These factors are important and influence how they continue to work in the complex and often sophisticated world of modern health and social care practice /education.

WHAT IS MEANT BY PROFESSIONALISM?

Professionalism is the characteristic thinking and behaviour of professionals, defined by the Chambers Dictionary (Allen 1994) as 'having the competence, expertise or conscientiousness of someone with professional training'. Friedson (1975) saw a profession as an occupation that has been given the right to control its own work. From this, a profession may be seen as autonomous, self-directing and embodying trustworthiness through adherence to ethics and knowledgeable skill. Common facets of professional behaviour are shared amongst the AHP group and have the following attributes that Kasar et al (1996) outlined for occupational therapy as an example:

■ Dependability.
■ Professional presentation.
■ Initiative.
■ Empathy.
■ Co-operation.
■ Organisation.

- Clinical reasoning.
- Supervisory process.
- Written and verbal communication (cited by Kaser and Muscan 2000, p. 44).

They go on to say that professional behaviours mature through a natural developmental process. Behaviours in this context can therefore be considered to form part of a sequential model of development described by Erikson (1982) as the life cycle completed. Leddy and Pepper (cited in Hood and Pepper 2002) described a similar model as the Conceptual Basis of Professional Nursing, as well as their own thoughts formulated as the professional development stage consisting of the following:

- Professional autonomy/independence.
- Professional responsibility/accountability.
- Professional attitudes.

The latter characteristics being:

- Educational background.
- Adherence to a code of ethics.
- Participation in professional organisations.
- Continuing education and competency.
- Self-regulation, communication and publication.
- Community service.
- Theory use and development.
- Evaluation and research involvement.

This said, Fish and Coles (1998) describe the professional as being under siege and propose that professionalism has eroded. This can be attributed to the following reasons:

- Increased lack of trustworthiness/confidence in the professional from society.
- Increased litigation being brought against the professional.
- Increased expectations of the professional from society be it the general public, government or professional bodies.
- Increased accountability and media highlighting malpractice (for example: The Kennedy Report 2001, which reported the Bristol children's autopsy scandal).

It is suggested that society is challenging professionals to justify and explain their professional judgements, actions and roles. To describe your practice as a 'hunch' or 'gut feeling' demeans the judgements and actions we take as therapists and is unsatisfactory to explain this to the general public. In a sense evidence-based practice, clinical guidelines and initiatives in therapy come into play to assist the professional to describe their roles and actions. Furthermore Fish and Coles (1998) present two views of professional practice:

- *The technical view* – 'professional practice as a basic matter of delivering a service to clients through a pre-determined set of clear-cut routines and behaviours' (p. 31).

■ *The professional artistry view* – 'professional activity is more akin to artistry, where only the principles can be pre-determined and practitioners may in practice and for good reason need to choose to go beyond them, just as good artists often go beyond or break artistic conventions in order to achieve an important effect . . . sees behaving professionally as being concerned with both means and ends' (p. 33).

With this in mind professional values are held in addition and form deeply held convictions of the practitioner's discipline and how these pertain to the rights of those served and the obligations of the individual practitioner. A value often has a moral, ethical, or philosophical basis concerning what is considered right, good, just or desirable. They are viewed as means of unifying the profession, providing a unique professional identity and promoting coherent practice.

PRE-REGISTRATION EDUCATION

One aim of reforming pre-registration medical education is to achieve a better balance between the emphasis on scientific knowledge and an enhancement of desirable professional attitudes: for example, reducing the core curriculum in physiology in order to increase learning opportunities in ethics. The education of AHPs in the UK has been prompted into reform also, by both public concern with examples of poor clinical performance and the demands of the Health Professions Council (HPC). A particular expectation is the development of desirable attitudes for professional practice and many curricula are now being restructured to show professional as well as clinical and academic outcomes. The teaching and learning of professional attitudes pose particular challenges, as attitudes are only indirectly revealed by our behaviours and actions and they cannot be altered purely by the receipt of knowledge. For example, whereas a student occupational therapist may learn how to carry out a dressing practice by a combination of learned facts and clinical experiences, they are likely to need a different set of learning experiences to gain the procedural skills involved in obtaining informed consent from a hospitalised Muslim patient for whom English is a third language. Moreover, the likelihood that personal and potentially stereotypical assumptions will be re-stimulated is greater in the latter than the former, and there is a much greater need to reflect on your own limits and abilities in the more complex situation. Thus professional development in healthcare education is becoming of increasing interest and the principles of adult learning, such as self-directed learning, reflective practice and problem-solving learning are being seen by many as bridges by which students will maximise relevant learning for professional experience (Maudsley and Strivens 2000).

Given the government's current concerns about the quality of public services such as health and social care and the important role of inter-professional working as a way of overcoming identified barriers, it comes as no surprise that inter-professional learning has become the focus of some new quality initiatives. However, healthcare education is often seen as being caught in a world of contested meaning between different groups (hospital, community, users, other professionals, the national health service and the university; to name but a few). Students have to struggle with these competing discourses during socialisation into their profession and the systems where they might work. To complicate this further, they find themselves being asked to develop differently depending on the setting they are in. It is common for students to hold contradictory values simultaneously but to utilise those which seem of most use in attaining the goals of the institution (Becker et al. 1961). In this way visible culture which is neither patient/user- nor student-centred will be a powerful barrier to the current goals of both public and professional leaders.

CODES OF ETHICS AND PROFESSIONAL CONDUCT

All AHPs have some kind of code/guidance governing the professionalism of their behaviour. The Code of Ethics and Professional Conduct for Occupational Therapists for example is produced by the professional body for and on behalf of the British Association of Occupational Therapists (BAOT), the central organisation for occupational therapists throughout the UK (College of Occupational Therapists [COT] 2000). The Health Act (1999) bestowed the status of a profession on occupational therapy along with other AHPs including physiotherapy, radiography and podiatry. This automatically carries the statutory requirement to regulate professional practice for the protection of all clients/service users/patients working with an AHP.

These codes of ethics state minimum standards for the professions and provide a set of principles that apply to all practitioners and students in practice. It is viewed by many as a public statement of the values and principles used in promoting and maintaining high standards of professional behaviour. More importantly in relation to litigation, the codes may be used evidentially and are written to apply to all individuals professionally engaged in practice and education of each respective profession. One clear statement for occupational therapists as an example states 'the code requires that practitioners discharge their duties and responsibilities in a professional, ethical and moral manner. It bestows no right on any person for its indiscriminate use of purposes other than those stated . . . ' (COT 2000, Section 1, p. 1). In this light, professional principles include important areas such as client autonomy and welfare, services to a client's personal/professional integrity, professional competence and standards.

One key way of achieving professional standards is through a process of continuing personal and professional development (CPD).

Professional and personal development

Professional development is defined as the activities which AHPs undertake to ensure that they provide an ever higher quality of service and strive for the highest level of attainment and/or responsibility in their work area. Personal development activities are defined as all other not strictly professional development activities, such as activities intended to equip therapists with skills or experience which can be beneficial to their practice and area of work, but not directly linked to it (Murray and Simpson 2000). The professional bodies subscribe to CPD as being the personal responsibility of all practitioners. Section 4 of the COT Code of Ethics for example advocates that members should . . . 'actively maintain and develop their personal professional competence . . . and shall base service delivery on accurate and current information in the interest of high quality care' (COT 2000, Section 5, p. 13).

One of the largest challenges facing all AHPs in modern day health and social care is the concept of CPD, often linked with discussions around the government's quality and clinical governance agenda. Recognising the importance of this concept is not new however as most professional bodies have incorporated personal and organisational accountability and responsibility for maintaining CPD for many years.

The Department of Health (DoH) 1998 suggests that CPD is a process of lifelong learning for all individuals and teams, meeting the needs of service users and delivering the health outcomes and healthcare priorities of the NHS thus enabling professionals to expand and fulfil their potential.

The inclusion of lifelong learning within this indicates clearly that our own professional journey is one that we undertake continuously for the rest of our professional lives. This notion has become one of the key components of the current government's intended overall framework to ensure high quality services are delivered in the health and social care services, especially through clinical governance.

In this context clinical governance is defined as:

> . . . a framework through which NHS organisations are accountable for continuously improving the quality of their services and safeguarding high standards of care by creating an environment in which excellence in clinical care can flourish.

> (DoH 1998, p. 4)

This important concept in health to drive quality has been subject to scrutiny by the AHP professional bodies to apply the principles within the parameters of their own professions, so for example the COT states:

> ... the basic principles of clinical governance relate to having an organised, integrated approach, thus safeguarding the quality of service provision to individual clients and the population. These principles apply equally to all occupational therapists whether they work in local authorities, health, criminal justice system, private hospitals, the voluntary sector, schools, industry or private practice. The College therefore stresses the need for occupational therapists to familiarise themselves with the principles and application of clinical governance in their own service areas. Similarly, therapists working in all areas are advised to familiarise themselves with social services quality initiatives, in order to assist joint quality activities. . . . occupational therapists should employ a range of quality activities in particular evidence-based practice . . . and continuing professional development . . .

> (COT 1999, p. 2)

Most professional bodies have published position statements, professional guidance and strategies on CPD. Many including the COT have incorporated CPD into the code of ethics and professional conduct (see above). A significant driver for this was the demise of the Council for Professions Supplementary to Medicine (CPSM), following the review of the Professions Supplementary to Medicine Act (1960). This led to a push to establish the Health Professions Council (HPC) as the new regulatory body in April 2002. Current debate indicates the likelihood of maintaining HPC registration being linked in some form to demonstrating and recording evidence of CPD (see Chapter 6). The mechanism for this has not yet been defined but linking evidence of CPD to the formal process of annual appraisals and/or individual performance reviews (IPR) seems a favourable option to evidence development.

Therapists need to take personal responsibility for their own professional development. However it is apparent that the government, professional bodies and academia also see CPD to mean more than simply updating clinical skills and knowledge. If it is to be understood as a process inherent in lifelong learning, it also may result in the development of a framework for continuous improvement in all aspects of practice and development. Essentially, five main paths of career development which professionals choose are specialisation, management, academia, research and private practice. All these provide new opportunities for therapists to deepen knowledge, skill and expertise in any of these chosen areas.

Career development

Most therapists still follow the traditional career pathway; that of starting professional work at a junior grade, before furthering their seniority through subsequent pay bands for progressively more experienced/specialist practitioners and AHP managers. Career pathways within modern health and to a lesser degree social care are far more fluid with new and contemporary opportunities constantly being introduced into the work environment, e.g. consultant therapists.

Therapists who progress into managerial positions however can activate management development at a range of levels from managing their own caseload to managing extensive staffing and other resources. Different mechanisms exist to upgrade management competencies and evidence-based practice/research have all become an essential part of any therapist's work and responsibilities. All research, be it informal evaluation of an aspect of intervention, outcome of an audit, or specific specialist research (part of or not part of an academic award), enriches the body of evidence on which all practitioners base their future intervention. Therapists who choose a teaching or academic career pathway contribute to professional development in many ways. These may include practising therapists who supervise practice placements for students, lecturer practitioner posts whereby therapists split their work between practice and teaching, and also full time formal academic teaching and facilitation within universities. This said, there is now an expectation that all therapists have a duty to undertake research activities to fulfil the statutory duty to keep clinical, managerial and academic skills up to date and therefore maintain their registration with the HPC.

RESEARCH AND PROFESSIONAL DEVELOPMENT

The concept of evidence-based practice is well established and understood (Chapter 9). If intervention is to be based on evidence however, individuals and teams must first become research active so that they can develop skills to apply and understand the latest research available. This is important as the latest research represents the most current evidence, not only from the UK and European context but also globally. However a substantial 'mind shift' has to occur when all therapists become producers of research rather than simply users of it; the process of research has to be owned actively at the coal face of practice rather than thought of as confined to specialist practitioners or academics. In this way all AHPs can contribute to the body of evidence to be used by others in the future (from within and outside their own professional groupings).

Although research activities as such cannot be properly described as a career pathway they are often combined with other activities; at present these are notably teaching or developing specialist knowledge and skill. It is worth noting that this might well change in the future with a mandatory requirement that every practitioner from the moment they graduate/qualify having a duty to embrace research activities throughout their career as part of their own CPD. Recent trends within AHPs indicate an increasing number of individuals embarking on higher degrees than ever before, notably at Masters, MPhil and PhD level, indicating greater interest in research at a more formalised level. Other developments in education for some AHPs to offer pre-registration programmes above a Bachelors level qualification (Postgrad Dip, MSc, even PhD) also enhances the number of people in practice with qualifications that indicate confidence in their research skills. It will be exciting over the next decade to see the effect that these developments have on the research profile of the AHPs who are as a group relatively new professions compared to medicine and nursing.

Developing specialist knowledge and the development of consultant therapists

One of the most significant developments in offering new career opportunities for AHPs is the concept of a highly qualified, advanced practitioner and specialist, who can act as, and is, officially recognised as a consultant therapist (Brown et al. 2003). This development was first included in the government's strategy for allied health professions called Meeting the Challenge (DoH 2000a). The DoH definitive definition of a consultant allied health professional is:

A consultant AHP is an expert in a specialist clinical field, bringing innovation, influence to clinical leadership and strategic direction in that particular field for the benefit of patients. The consultant will play a pivotal role in the integration of research evidence into practice. Exceptional skills and advanced levels of clinical judgement, knowledge and experience will underpin and promote the delivery of the clinical governance agenda. This will be by enhancing quality in areas of assessment, diagnosis, management and evaluation, delivering improved outcomes for patients and extending the parameters of the specialism.

(DoH 2000a, p. 2)

In addition the government's vision for this new development is specified in the following DoH statement:

Consultant posts provide the opportunity to retain clinical excellence and mature skills within the service. They will sit within a range of models of practice and service configuration. While the focus of the consultant posts will be the delivery and practice of clinical care, the development of more detailed job descriptions will be undertaken at local level, tailored to meet local needs and based on local circumstances. This ensures that AHPs can develop through a range of opportunities and routes, either as specialists or generalist practitioners to consultant level in the acute, community and intermediate care settings. This approach gives services the flexibility to meet their specific needs within the local community.

(DoH 2000a, p. 6)

At the time of writing the establishment of these posts is still relatively new, so the impact of these post-holders on the quality of professional service in the NHS is difficult to assess. The substantive pay scales for these positions compared with senior level practice, management and academic posts would suggest that this initiative will prove to be popular amongst potential applicants. These posts certainly mark a definitive move in recognising the professionalism of allied health practitioners.

WORKING WITHIN PROFESSIONAL BOUNDARIES

Over the past 20 years, multi-disciplinary and multi-agency teams have been a central component of health and social care services in the UK, and in particular in mental health policy (DoH 1995, 1999, Department of Health and Social Services 1975). The aspirations for these teams was that they would 'provide a service in which the boundaries between primary healthcare, secondary healthcare and social care do not form barriers seen from the perspective of the service user' (DoH 1990, p. 16). In policy terms, agency and professional boundaries were perceived as barriers; teams were the chosen method of overcoming them.

The imperative to collaborate across service and professional boundaries in order effectively to tackle perceived inequities in service delivery is clear. In addition to the greater flexibility available to the new Primary Care Trusts (England and equivalents in other UK nations: see Chapter 1, Figure 1.2), the local authorities and NHS organisations are also able to pool budgets and integrate services for some specific groups of people. This said, it is clear that there are still some professional and organisational barriers which can inhibit or facilitate joint service commissioning. An important aspect of 'being professional' for the AHPs will be to address such barriers so for example greater integration across the primary care/local authority divide is achieved.

It may be that some professional groups are more able than others to adapt to the new imperatives to work flexibly and in collaboration with others. Occupational therapists for example, with a traditional role in both health and social services, are key in developing closer, flexible working relationships between the services of these organisations without threatening the core professional identity. Whilst the government has allowed GPs in particular to take the lead in the governance of primary care groups, this will not necessarily be the case with PCTs and their other UK equivalents. Here AHPs and nurses are likely to take a more prominent role and this may help to boost the overall objectives of creating better integrated services and closer inter-professional working.

The overcoming of professional boundaries has become one of the key goals of health and social services policy in the UK in the past 7 years. The impact of this has been greatly experienced by all health and social care professionals with a move towards cross boundary working at both uniprofessional and inter-professional levels, thus pushing professional relationships to new heights. It is important to note that boundaries between agencies and professionals may often come into being through differences in organisational structures and values (Stantham 2000), and through professional elitist beliefs (see Chapter 5). In turn they may be inculcated into individuals through in-service training and sustained patterns of socialisation (Peck and Norman 1999, cited in Sale 2000), and often underpinned by being enacted in discrete physical spaces. Although in policy terms they may be an obstacle to be overcome (DoH 2000b), they can simultaneously be conceptualised as crucial to making individuals feel secure in their work.

Maintaining professional boundaries poses a particular challenge for most professions and organisations due to unclear task definitions. But in modern days health and social care communities, working in partnership with others whilst maintaining and protecting professional identity is in itself viewed as having a true professional attitude to work. It is often within inter-professional working that issues around boundaries are negotiated, through the modification of roles and relationships within teams and by the response of these teams to demands from outside such as service users, carers, national policy and even our own professional vision.

The publication of the White Paper, The New NHS: Modern, Dependable (DoH 1997) within the first year of the incoming Labour Government, formally signalled the demise of the old 'internal market' created under the Conservatives and the perceived power base of the 'medical model' in determining how health services were shaped and made available to the public. This was through the creation of a system based on 'the external market' driven equally by a more 'social model of care' based on the holistic needs of service users rather than how their needs were perceived by medical practitioners. This shift provided an opportunity for the AHPs to have a more equal influence on the development of a new health and social care model within the UK. However, the agenda set out in the White Paper was much more radical than the simple fulfilment of an election pledge to abolish a two tier service. It emphasised the role of the NHS, in partnership with local authority and other statutory organisations, in improving health; set out a renewed commitment to equity of access and service provision; and tackled the variable quality of certain aspects of the agenda through new systems of 'clinical governance'.

These changes in structural and decision-making systems in health and social care are in synthesis with the AHP agenda for consolidating their professionalism in practice. Changes in recent times have both facilitated the development of true professional practice for the AHP group and allowed them to impact their expertise and thinking on the health and social care concepts, policy and implementation.

CONCLUSION

AHPs have had to adapt to a changing world that has required self-regulation, greater responsibility and accountability. The professions could be seen as passing through a developmental process in which they have had to grow up to meet the more complex demands of modern times.

Reflective questions:

■ Using the list of professional attributes outlined by Kaser and Muscan (2000), think through an aspect of your everyday practice. How do these attributes link to this aspect of your work? What influences this?

■ Consider the different career options of senior practitioner, manager, consultant therapist or university AHP educator: How do these contribute to the overall professional development of your discipline? What options are available to you? How might each affect your professional skills? How do these link with current government agendas?

REFERENCES

Allen R (ed.) 1994 *Chambers encyclopaedic English dictionary*. Chambers, Edinburgh.

Becker HS, Geer B, Hughes E, Strauss A 1961 *Boys in white; student culture in medical school*. University of Chicago Press, Chicago.

Brown G, Esdaile SA, Ryan S 2003 *Advanced healthcare practitioner*. Butterworth Heinemann, Oxford.

College of Occupational Therapists 1999 *Position Statement on Clinical Governance*. College of Occupational Therapists, London.

College of Occupational Therapists 2000 *The Code of Ethics and Professional Conduct*. College of Occupational Therapists, London.

Department of Health and Social Services 1975 *Better services for the mentally ill*. Cmnd 6239. HMSO, London.

Department of Health 1990 *Community care in the next decade and beyond*. HMSO, London.

Department of Health 1995 *Building bridges*. HMSO, London.

Department of Health 1997 *The new NHS: modern, dependable*. HMSO, London.

Department of Health 1998 *A first class service – quality in the NHS*. HMSO, London.

Department of Health 1999 *National Service Framework for Mental Health*. HMSO, London.

Department of Health 2000a *A strategy for the allied health professions*. Meeting the Challenge. HMSO, London.

Department of Health 2000b *The NHS Plan: a plan for investment, a plan for reform*. Cmnd 4880. HMSO, London

Erikson E 1982 *Eric Erikson's 8 stages of psychosocial development*. Online. Available: http://web.cortland.edu/andersmd/ERIK/bio.HTML. 8 December 2003.

Fish D, Coles C 1998 *Developing professional judgements in healthcare: learning through critical appreciation of practice*. Butterworth Heinemann, Oxford.

Friedson E 1975 *Profession of medicine: a study of the sociology of applied knowledge*. Dodd, Mead and Co, New York.

Health Act 1999 Stationery Office, London.

Hood L, Pepper JM 2002 *Conceptual basis of professional nursing*. Lippincott Williams and Wilkins, Baltimore.

Kasar J, Muscan ME 2000 A conceptual model of development of professional behaviours in occupational therapists. *Canadian Journal of Occupational Therapy* 67(1): 42–50.

Kasar J, Clark N, Watson D, Pfister S 1996 *Professional development assessment*. Unpublished document.

Kennedy Report 2001 *The inquiry into the management of care of children receiving complex heart surgery at Bristol Royal Infirmary: Final report*. Online. Available: http://www.bristol-inquiry.org.uk/final_report/index.htm accesses 28 November 2003.

Maudsley G, Strivens J 2000 Promoting professional knowledge, experiential learning and critical thinking of medical students. *Journal of Medical Education* 34: 535–544.

Murray E, Simpson J 2000 *Professional development and management for therapists*. Blackwell Science, Oxford.

Professions Supplementary to Medicine Act 1960 HMSO, London.

Sale D 2000 *Quality assurance: a pathway to excellence*. Macmillan, London.

Stantham D 2000 Guest editorial: partnership between health and social care. *Health and Social Care in the Community* 8: 87–89.

RECOMMENDED READING

Allsop A 2002 Portfolios: portraits of our professional lives. *British Journal of Occupational Therapy* 65(5): 201–206.

Bishop V 1998 *Clinical supervision in practice*. Macmillan Press, London.

College of Occupational Therapists 1998 *Clinical governance: a position statement*. College of Occupational Therapists, London.

College of Occupational Therapists 2002 Position statement on lifelong learning, London. *British Journal of Occupational Therapy* 65(5): 198–200.

Commission for Health Improvement 2003 *About CHI*.
Online. Available:
http://www.chi.nhs.uk
13 January 2004.

Department of Health 1990 *Community care in the next decade and beyond.* HMSO, London.

Department of Health 1995 *Building bridges.* HMSO, London.

Department of Health 1999 *National service framework for mental health.* HMSO, London.

Department of Health 2000 *The NHS Plan: a plan for investment, a plan for reform.* Cmnd 4880. HMSO, London.

Newell R 2003 *Clinical governance.*
Online. Available:
http://www.doh.gov.uk/governance/
10 January 2004.

Simpson J 1998 How good is your documentation. *Physiotherapy* 84(10): 469–471.

PART 2 Development of the professions and individual practitioner

Conclusion

Lyn Westcott and Teena J. Clouston

This second part of the book has discussed some important areas that focus on issues of professionalism within the contexts of health and social care.

Understanding health and social care professions from sociological perspectives (Chapter 4), helped the reader to appreciate the broader concept of professionalism and how this might link to your identity as an AHP. It also explored how different professional groups fit into the wider concept of society and the legislative framework that now surrounds the AHP group. This should have provided a framework to understand your professionalism and how this might impact on your behaviour and attitudes to practice.

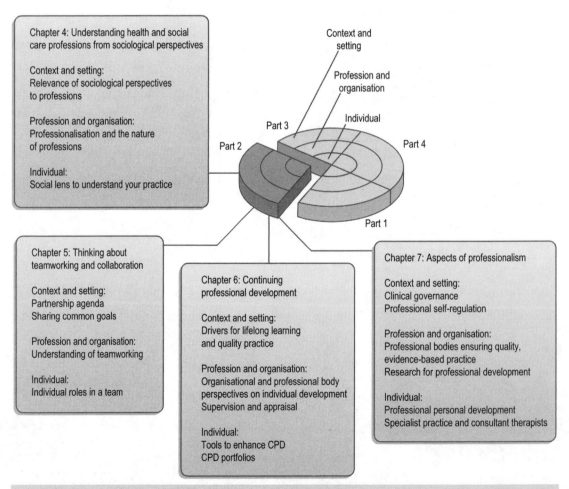

Part 2 Summary Development of the professions and individual practitioner

Thinking about teamworking and collaboration (Chapter 5), may have challenged your basic understanding of teams in health and social care contexts. It set out to help you think through your own role as a team member and how that team might best work in the current climate affecting AHP practice.

Continuing professional development (Chapter 6), discussed the legislative and practical application of this important foundation to professional practice. This chapter should have helped you think through some practical ideas to recognise and action a range of activities that will enhance your professional growth over time.

Aspects of professionalism (Chapter 7) discussed broad legislative concepts impacting on professionalism and newer pathways being created to develop individual practice. This is linked to the agenda for change and self-regulation and can be seen as enhancing the professional standing of AHPs.

The figure on page 114 provides a brief summary of key issues considered throughout Part 2, highlighting their relevance to the professions and how this links to the individual practitioner and organisations in which they work.

PART 3 Professional influences on practice

Introduction

Lyn Westcott and Teena J. Clouston

This third part of the book sets out to examine some important forces that shape contemporary practice for AHPs. These areas are:

- Quality agenda in health and social care (Chapter 8).
- How to be an evidence-based practitioner (Chapter 9).
- Audit in AHP practice (Chapter 10).
- Legal influences on practice (Chapter 11).

To help you make sense of your thinking and understanding of these influential issues, you may find it helpful to consider how these impact on your practice from three perspectives.

As an individual allied health practitioner (AHP), you may be aware of elements of these issues and how they impact on your practice. You may not, however, have considered each in detail as distinct entities. The chapters in this part of the book all have some focus on the individual to help you make sense of these areas in practice.

At a professional and organisational level all these topics have significant influence to bear on the understanding and mechanics of health and social care delivery. Indeed these areas have been pivotal in shaping recent developments in the structure of service provision.

The issues discussed in this part of the book have all emerged from a need for accountability to the public sector being bound to the public expectation of high standards in an effective, efficient, accessible health and social care system. This in turn reflects the government philosophy of and emphasis on offering the best possible service within finite resources.

In order to make sense of Part 3, you are advised to bear in mind the three domains of context and setting, professional and organisation and individual practice. This will help you understand why the text is relevant to you. These themes are revisited within the conclusion and summary found at the end of Part 3, which includes an illustration of key areas within each chapter under these headings.

The quality agenda in health and social care

Gwilym Wyn Roberts

LEARNING OUTCOMES

- To identify defining moments in the development of the quality agenda.
- To gain an understanding of key quality issues.
- To consider the relevance of quality to AHP practice.
- To reflect on the importance of service user involvement.

INTRODUCTION

The definition of 'quality' has been built on from the idea put forward by the World Health Organization (WHO), where quality was described as encapsulating the following four elements:

1. Professional Management (technical quality).
2. Resources (efficiency).
3. Risk Management.
4. Satisfaction of patients with the service provided.

(WHO 1986)

Delivering an excellent service user/patient-centred health and social care service has been an important factor in the UK's government quality agenda. In his report following the Bristol Inquiry, Sir Ian Kennedy set out a vision and a challenge for the future of the National Health Service (NHS) to build a new culture; one of trust not blame, with greater partnership between patients and professionals, clear lines of accountability, openness about mistakes, services designed from patients' points of view and where safety for patients always comes first (Kennedy Report 2001). Alan Milburn, the then Minister for Health, responded by saying that the government did not underestimate the extent of Kennedy's ambition, but it was a challenge they accepted. The Bristol Inquiry is seen by many as a vital turning point for the NHS, with good coming out of tragedy.

THE BRISTOL INQUIRY (THE KENNEDY REPORT)

Some events can be classified as defining moments; they change the ways in which people see and respond to their environment. The disaster at Bristol Royal Infirmary was a defining moment for health and social care in the UK. This was because parents who had been bereaved following unsuccessful heart surgery on their babies and young children, discovered that body parts had been retained without permission at autopsy. This caused an understandable scandal with the media highlighting the distress of families and castigating the medical services for unethical practice. The consequent inquiry into services provided by the paediatric cardiac surgical team between 1984 and 1995 has become a watershed in the development of UK health and social care services. The foreword to the Bristol Inquiry report summarised the nature of the disaster in the following way:

> There were failings both of organisations and people. Some children and their parents were failed. Some parents suffered the loss of a child when it should not have happened. A tragedy took place. But it was a tragedy born of high hopes and ambitions, and peopled by dedicated, hard working people. The hopes were too high; the ambitions too ambitious. Bristol simply overreached itself. Many patients, children and adults benefited; too many children did not. Too many children died.
>
> (Kennedy Report, 2001 p. 1)

The report suggested that there was an organisational failure of foresight based on a series of systematic and communication failures that contributed to oversight of an 'incubating' hazard which ultimately led to disaster. The recommendation of the Kennedy report provided a major stimulus to the modernisation programme and especially of governance in health and social care which aimed to restore public confidence and create trusting organisations. Whilst it is premature to evaluate the impact of the changes, many would argue that there is little evidence at present to indicate that they will improve the quality of professional decision making and the safety of users or enhance user and public confidence in the NHS and other public services.

Nonetheless, the Bristol Inquiry is a watershed because it marked a major change in the government's relationship with the professions in general and in particular the medical profession. It emerged that the government was no longer willing to unconditionally trust the medical profession to regulate itself and provide a uniform standard of care. Variations in the standard of care were now considered to be totally unacceptable. Clinical autonomy, the professional control of decision making and management of risk, which had so conspicuously failed at Bristol, has been replaced by clinical governance, the external inspection of decision making and management of risk.

For the allied health professions (AHPs), the recommendation of the Bristol Inquiry provided a major stimulus to the modernisation programme for health and social care which aimed to restore public confidence and create a high-trust organisation. The modernisation agenda is designed to reverse the perceived decline in public confidence in services such as the NHS and restore trust in services and those professionals who deliver them. The recommendations are intended to contribute directly to improving confidence by enhancing public involvement through empowerment and ensuring respect and honesty for users and carers and indirectly by developing management and leadership and creating a culture of safety.

THE QUALITY AGENDA

Although much of the NHS is deemed as excellent by any standards, Kennedy highlighted failure of communication, lack of leadership, paternalism, a club culture and a failure to put patients at the centre of care. Failings at Bristol resulted in death of and damage to a number of very young children; as a result, separate to the Kennedy report, but related to it, the Labour Government put forward radical new arrangements.

Previously the Department of Health (DoH) was both the regulator and the headquarters for the NHS. Its style and approach was likened to a mid 20th century nationalised industry. A need was therefore identified for change that would provide objective and creative support to adapt the NHS to 21st century ideals and that were innovative and responsive to patients' needs. This vision included the relocation of resources and responsibilities to front-line services (for example, through primary care trusts [PCTs] and NHS trusts), and a range of independent advice and controls. These included:

- National Service Frameworks (NSFs) that set standards for key areas of treatment.
- The National Institute for Clinical Excellence (NICE) that provides evidence-based standards.
- The Citizen's Council that provides advice to NICE on the values inherent in its decisions and its guidance on treatments.
- The Healthcare Commission or Commission for Healthcare Audit and Inspection (CHAI) and the Social Care Inspection Commission that inspect and should ensure effective quality assurance and improvement mechanisms.
- The National Patient Safety Agency that provides a single national system for reporting and analysis of adverse events and near misses and ensures effective learning takes place to make the NHS a safer place for patients.
- The National Clinical Assessment Authority that helps NHS employers assess identified poorly performing doctors.
- A council for the quality of healthcare professionals – the Health Professions Council (HPC) replaced the former Council for Professions Supplementary to Medicine (CPSM) with the purpose of strengthening professional self-regulation (HPC 2003).
- The Commission for Patient and Public Involvement in Health sets standards and provides training and guidance for effective community involvement.
- Continuing improvement will be supported by the Modernisation Agency, Leadership Centre and NHS University in spreading good practice and developing leadership.

All these bodies collectively have a responsibility to ensure quality services and public safety and work with clinical professions to ensure that all allied health professionals, doctors, nurses and all healthcare workers are supported to provide the highest quality care and be held accountable.

Ultimately, however, service user empowerment and involvement has been highlighted as a cornerstone in quality and consequently the following organisations and strategies have developed:

- The National Knowledge Service provides information to patients on how different local services compare.
- The Patient Advice and Liaison Service (PALS) found in every trust, assists patients/service users to access and manage information.
- The Expert Patient Programme supports clinician/patient partnerships.
- A new complaints procedure has also been introduced and data on clinical performance of consultants and medical teams published to be more accessible.

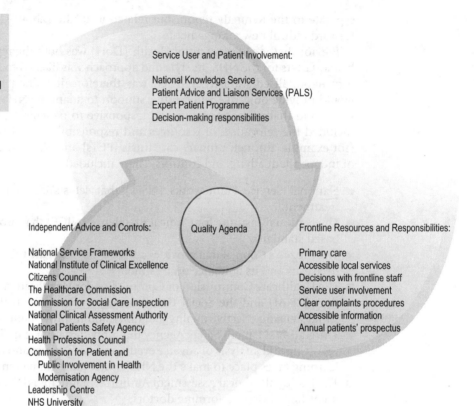

Figure 8.1
The impacts of the quality agenda on health and social care.

From 2005 electronic patient records will make it easier to facilitate this process.

■ PCTs and Trusts will be required to produce an annual 'patient prospectus', showing the amount and impact of public involvement.

■ Stringent guidelines on sharing information with patients and with young children's parents have been developed to enhance user involvement through provision of more information and greater say over local services and who provides their care (see Figure 8.1).

CLINICAL GOVERNANCE

The new vision for the NHS identified clinical governance as a modern term for what was previously known as quality assurance. Following the impact of some very high profile critical incidents such as the Bristol Inquiry, the emphasis was clearly put on quality, financial responsibility, good practice, professional self-regulation and assessing and minimising risks. Clinical governance is often described as a system through which the NHS organisation is made accountable for continuously improving the quality of their services and safe guarding high standards of care by creating an environment in which excellence in clinical care will flourish (Dewar 1999).

Clinical governance encapsulates the steps and procedures adopted by the NHS to ensure that service users receive the highest possible quality of care, including a patient-centred approach, accountability for quality, high standards and safety to enable improvement in patient services and care. The Chief Medical Officer Sir Liam Donaldson defined clinical governance as 'a system through which NHS organisations are accountable for continuously improving the quality of their services and safeguarding high standards of care, by creating an environment in which clinical excellence will flourish'. Harrison and van Zwanenberg (1998, p. 11) defined it as 'a powerful, new and comprehensive mechanism for ensuring that high quality standards of clinical care are maintained throughout the NHS and that quality of services is continuously improved'.

The agenda for quality improvement set out in the White Paper – A First Class Service: Quality in the New NHS (DoH 1998a) provided both an opportunity and a challenge for every health professional and manager. This white paper arose from another equally important one namely The New NHS: Modern, Dependable (1997). Both papers identified quality as a key issue in modernising the NHS. At the heart of this agenda is a requirement for NHS organisations to seek to improve and assure quality through a system of clinical governance. Backed by a statutory duty of quality, which balances existing financial duties, clinical governance is the main vehicle driving improvements in the quality of NHS care. The basic components are a coherent approach to quality improvement, clear lines of accountability for clinical quality systems and effective processes for identifying and managing risk and addressing poor performance. Above all though, clinical governance is about the culture of NHS organisations. A culture where openness and participation are encouraged, where education and research are properly valued, where people learn from failures and blame is the exception rather than the rule, and where good practice and new approaches are freely shared and willingly received (Swage 2000).

The principles of clinical governance according to the NHS Executive (1999) are:

- Clear lines of responsibility and accountability for the overall quality of clinical care.
- A comprehensive programme of quality improvement systems (including clinical audit, supporting evidence-based practice, implementing clinical standards and guidelines, workforce planning and development).
- Education and training plans.
- Clear policies aimed at management of risk.
- Integrated procedures for all professional groups to identify and remedy poor performance.

In response to this Swage (2000) reported that the success criteria in clinical governance (as viewed by the London Regional Office of the NHS Executive) to monitor and ensure that systems are functioning appropriately (including both processes and outcome measures) are:

- Appropriate cultural/environmental conditions.
- Staff and organisational development.
- General overview and bringing together.
- Clinical audit.

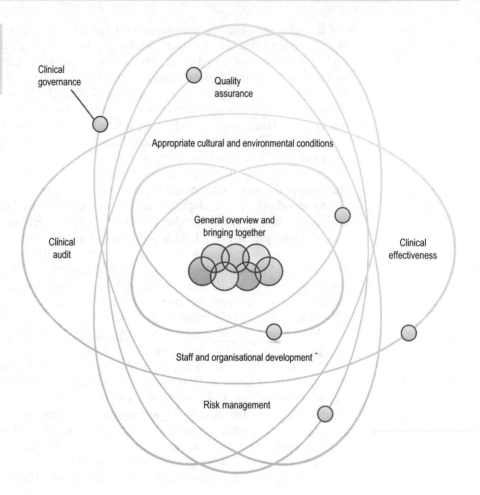

Figure 8.2
Success criteria
for clinical
governance.

■ Clinical risk management.
■ Clinical effectiveness.
■ Quality assurance.

(See Figure 8.2.)

Professional and statutory bodies play an important role in setting and promoting standards, but shifting the focus towards quality also required practitioners to accept responsibility for developing and maintaining standards within their local NHS organisations. For this reason the government required every NHS Trust to embrace the concept of clinical governance so that quality was put at the core, both of their responsibilities as organisations and of each of their staff as individual professionals.

In this context, a quality organisation would be expected to ensure the following:

■ Quality improvement processes (for example clinical audit) are in place and integrated with the quality programme for the organisation as a whole.
■ Leadership skills are developed at clinical team level.
■ Evidence-based practice is in day to day use with infrastructure to support it.

- Good practice ideas and innovations (which have been evaluated) are systematically disseminated within and outside the organisation.
- Clinical risk reduction programmes of a high standard are in place.
- Adverse events are detected, openly investigated and the lessons learned promptly applied.
- Lessons for clinical practice are systematically learned from complaints made by patients/service users.
- Problems of poor clinical performance are recognised at an early stage and dealt with to prevent harm to patients.
- All professional development programmes reflect the principles of clinical governance.
- Quality of data collected to monitor clinical care is itself of a high standard.
- Most importantly chief executives of trusts are now expected to ensure that there are appropriate local arrangements to give them and the NHS Trust Board firm assurances that their responsibilities for quality are being met, including equity in providing resources for continuing professional development of all its employees.

CLINICAL EFFECTIVENESS

The clinical effectiveness framework was set up to ensure that clinical standards were being met and that processes were in place to ensure continuous improvement. In addition it also advocated the setting up of clear national standards with responsibility for delivery being taken locally and backed by consistent monitoring arrangements. This devolution of responsibility was matched with accountability necessitated in a national public service such as the NHS (Sale 2000). In line with this national standards were developed through national service frameworks as well as through the national institute of clinical excellence (NICE). The standards were set for major areas of care and disease groups, to the extent that NICE became a special health authority in 1999. In addition the Commission for Health Improvement (CHI now called CHAI or the Healthcare Commission) was set up to monitor the quality of clinical services at local level to tackle shortcomings. What was significant about CHI was its ability to intervene if necessary where problems were identified. CHI would also be expected to ensure that healthcare organisations were able to fulfil their responsibilities to clinical governance (CHI 2003).

BEST VALUE

'Best value' was introduced in 2001, and was seen as the government's vision for improving the quality of local government services. Best value is defined in the Local Government Act 1999 as 'securing continuous improvement in the exercise of all functions undertaken by the authority, whether statutory or not, having regard to a combination of economy, efficiency and effectiveness'. It is seen as a process which aims clearly to achieve improvements to a given service so that the service itself is delivered to its customers in the most efficient and effective way possible. Many would see this as a desirable objective for any service, and one could argue that it is good management practice to ensure that procedures are already in place to routinely achieve this. The government published a

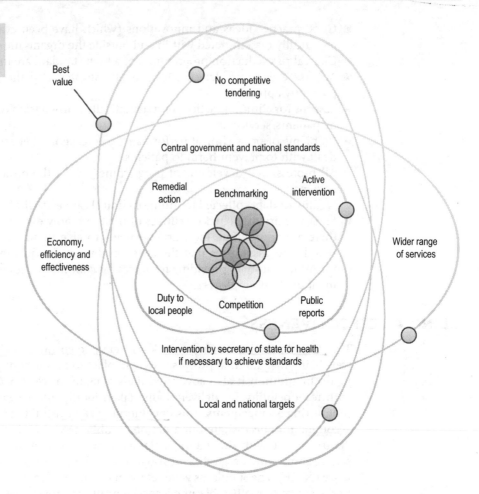

Figure 8.3
12 principles of best value.

Best value

No competitive tendering

Central government and national standards

Remedial action

Benchmarking

Active intervention

Economy, efficiency and effectiveness

Wider range of services

Duty to local people

Competition

Public reports

Intervention by secretary of state for health if necessary to achieve standards

Local and national targets

provisional list of 12 key principles of best value in June 1997 (see Figure 8.3). These were later reproduced in the English and Welsh Green Papers Modernising Local Government: Improving Local Services through Best Value (DoH 1998b) and Modernising Local Government in Wales: Improving Local Services through Best Value (Welsh Assembly Government 1998).

The key element in best value is the evaluation of performance management in the form of service reviews annually and over a 5-year rolling cycle (DoH 1999a). Evaluation in this context includes local performance plans and inspections evaluating effectiveness of the service, comparing local performance with other councils, consulting with the service users and community for a better service and creating a certain amount of competitiveness between the different councils. Best value inspections previously from the Audit Commission and Social Services Inspectorate and now the Commission for Social Care Inspection (CSCI) ensure that best value standards and practice are in place, monitored through the annual and 5-yearly reviews. Inspection reports, published by the Commission give each council a star rating based on performance, ranging from no stars for poor performance to three stars for excellent performance. The reports also provide an assessment of whether performance is likely to improve.

However, the best value process goes further by stressing the importance of the following areas of social care and in particular:

- Consulting with those who use the service to identify the priorities for the users.
- Consulting with those who work in the service at all levels to determine what does and what does not work well and to obtain innovative ideas about the way improvements could be made.
- Comparing/benchmarking the performance of the service against any local or national indicators which may be available.
- Challenging existing processes to ascertain if a service could be provided in a better way.
- Recommending options for change in line with the results of consultation. Changes could range from small improvements to processes, to a major reconfiguration of a service. In some circumstances the move to an alternative service provider might be considered, but only if it can be demonstrated that this might lead to improved value for money.
- Competing wherever practical.

Local government organisations have been required to implement best value since it became enshrined in law in 2000.

PROFESSIONAL SELF-REGULATION

Professional self-regulation is a process which provides clinicians with the opportunity to help set standards. It is understood that society needs to be confident that professional bodies will exercise rigorous self-regulation over the standards and conduct of health professionals and will act promptly and openly when things go wrong. The government is expected to commit to working with professional bodies and professional regulatory bodies to ensure that professional self-regulation keeps pace with public expectations and is more open and accountable. As an example, a modernised regulatory system will play a fuller part in the early identification of possible lapses in clinical quality (DoH 2001a).

In addition The Health Act 1999 stated that the purpose of self-regulation was to establish a countrywide, professionally set, independent standard of training, conduct and competence for each profession for the protection of the public and the guidance of employers. This is underpinned by personal accountability of practitioners for maintaining safe and effective practice, wherever they are employed and to include effective measures to deal with individuals whose continuing practice represents an unacceptable risk to the public or otherwise renders them unfit to be a registered member of the profession.

The Health Act 1999 also introduced a 'duty of care' on NHS Trusts, PCTs and health authorities. The original commission for health improvement (CHI), now the Commission for Healthcare Audit and Inspection was also set up to oversee the implementation of that duty into practice through clinical governance. The government, through the Health Act has been able to confirm the importance of self-regulation in its plan by stating 'professional self-regulation must remain an essential element in the delivery of quality patient services . . . the government will continue to work with the professions, the regulatory bodies, the NHS and patient representative groups to strengthen the existing systems of professional self-regulation by ensuring they are open, responsive and publicly accountable' (National Consumer Council [NCC] 1999). The NCC goes on to note 'recent events have dented public confidence in the quality of care provided by the NHS. The challenge for the professions is to demonstrate that professional self-regulation can continue to enjoy public confidence'. One tool in harnessing this confidence is by assuring quality service provision through the knowledge and skill of staff.

The government gave notice of its plans for lifelong learning in its pre-election manifesto. Its vision for a learning society was first published in the Learning to Succeed White Paper in 1999 and its health service circular (HSC) (DoH 1999b, DoH 2001b). Contemporaneously, both the Modernising Social Services (DoH 1998c) and A First Class Service: Quality in the NHS (DoH 1997) White Papers attached great importance to continuing professional development (CPD) for all staff whether qualified or unqualified. A First Class Service set out a package of proposals to support the delivery of more consistent and higher quality level of care to patients. The main elements of A First Class Service were:

- Arrangements for setting clear national standards through NSFs and NICE.
- Mechanisms for ensuring local delivery of high quality clinical services through clinical governance reinforced by a new statutory duty of quality and supported by programmes of lifelong learning and local delivery of professional self-regulation.
- Effective systems of monitoring delivery of quality standards, in the form of a new statutory Commission for Health Improvement (CHI) and an NHS Performance assessment Framework, together with the first survey of patients and user experience.

The College of Occupational Therapists (COT 2003a) stated that the evidence of professional competence should be attained by providing a continuing professional development portfolio. In addition they recommended that it is the responsibility of the individual staff member to maintain and defend their continued capability. This applies to all AHPs and as such you must be able to justify the decisions you make to undertake a treatment activity and explain your competence to use it. CPD is applicable to all therapists, support workers, assistants and technicians, administration staff, volunteers and managers.

CPD is not only about formal learning (COT 2003b); it is about work-based learning and benefit to users/patients. The government acknowledges the role of professional bodies in ensuring competence to practise. With this acknowledgement comes individual accountability as CPD becomes a statutory requirement.

CONCLUSION

Quality in health and social care is a complex term with seemingly diverse meanings in the health and social care arenas. However, there are strong commonalities between clinical governance and best value that allow a shared value system to exist and provide a basis for partnerships at organisational, professional and individual levels. These include lifelong learning, continuous professional development, professional self-regulation, individual responsibility, external moderation and patient/service user involvement. In simple terms, quality is everyone's responsibility.

REFERENCES

COT 2003a Continuing professional development: Why now?
Online. Available:
http://www.cot.co.uk/members/cpd/examples/whynow.asp
1 Aug 2003.

COT 2003b CPD. *Where does CPD fit?*
Online. Available:
http://www.cot.co.uk/members/cpd/examples/where.asp
1 Aug 2003.

Commission for Health Improvement 2003 *About CHI.*
Online. Available:
http://www.chi.nhs.uk
1 Aug 2003.

Department of Health 1997 *The new NHS: modern, dependable.* Department of Health, London.

Department of Health 1998a *A first class service: quality in the new NHS.* Department of Health, London.

Department of Health 1998b *Modernising local government: improving local services through best value.* Department of Health, London.

Department of Health 1998c *Modernising social services.* Department of Health, London.

Department of Health 1999a *A new approach to social services performance.* Department of Health, London.

Department of Health 1999b *Continuing professional development: quality in the new NHS,* HSC 99/154 Department of Health, London.

Department of Health 2001a *Establishing the new Health Professions Council.* Department of Health, London.

Department of Health 2001b *Working together, learning together. A framework for lifelong learning in the NHS.*
Online. Available:
http://www.dh.gov.uk/Home/fs/en
2 April 2004.

Dewar S 1999 *Clinical governance under construction.* Kings Fund, London.

Harrison J, van Zwanenberg T 1998 *GP tomorrow.* Radcliffe Medical Press, Oxford.

Health Act 1999 HMSO, London.

Health Professions Council 2003 *About us.*
Online: Available
http://www.hpc-uk.org/doc/about-us.htm
1 Aug 2003.

Kennedy Report 2001 *Learning from Bristol: the report of the public inquiry into children's heart surgery at The Bristol Royal Infirmary* 1984–1995. Command Paper CM 5207, 2001. The Stationery Office, London.

Local Government Act 1999 HMSO, London.

National Consumer Council 1999 *Self-regulation of professionals in healthcare.* London National Consumers Council, London.

NHS Executive 1999 *Primary care – clinical governance.*
Online. Available:
http://www.doh.gov.uk/pricare/clingov.htm
1 Aug 2003.

Sale D 2000 *Quality assurance: a pathway to excellence.* Macmillan Press, London.

Swage T 2000 *Clinical governance in healthcare practice.* Oxford Reed, London.

Welsh Assembly Government 1998 *Modernising local government in Wales: improving local services through best value.* Welsh Assembly Government, Cardiff.

World Health Organization 1986 *Ottawa Charter for health promotion.* Department of National Health and Welfare, Ottawa.

RECOMMENDED READING

Brown G, Esdaile SA, Ryan SE 2003 *Becoming an advanced healthcare practitioner*. Butterworth Heinemann, London.
Department of Health 1998 *Partnership in action*. Department of Health, London.

9 How to be an evidence-based practitioner

Linda Lovelock

LEARNING OUTCOMES

After reading this chapter you will be able to:
- Explain what is meant by evidence-based practice.
- Understand the different types of evidence available.
- Evaluate the skills required to be an evidence-based practitioner.

INTRODUCTION

The previous chapters in this book have outlined the current context and climate in which health and social care services are delivered. One very important consequence of the changes in public attitude and government policy is that we must now be able to justify our choice of interventions to the people who employ us and, more importantly, to the people who receive a service from us. Primarily this is by using the available evidence regarding the effectiveness, appropriateness and acceptability of selected treatments and interventions. However, it also requires a more explicit awareness of the clinical reasoning processes that we use and a willingness to share this with our patients and clients.

This chapter aims to explain what is meant by evidence-based practice and provide a practical introduction to becoming an evidence-based practitioner. It explores the different types of evidence available, considers how to access evidence and how to develop and enhance skills of critical analysis.

WHAT IS EVIDENCE-BASED PRACTICE?

The term evidence-based medicine was first coined to consider intervention by doctors, but this was subsequently broadened to encompass other health professionals and called evidence-based practice. More recent writers have applied it to specific areas such as rehabilitation and also attempted to incorporate the entire health and social care system. The definitions highlighted in Example 9.1 may suggest subtle differences in approach, but they are essentially saying the same thing. That is, to be an evidenced-based practitioner, we should be familiar with the most recent evidence about the effectiveness of the interventions we use and moreover use that knowledge, together with clinical judgement, to work with the patient, user or client.

Example 9.1

'Evidence-based medicine is the conscientious, explicit and judicious use of current best evidence in making decisions about the care of individual patients. The practice of evidence-based medicine means integrating individual clinical expertise with the best available external clinical evidence from systematic research' (Sackett et al. 1996, p. 71).

'Evidence-based clinical practice is an approach to decision making in which the clinician uses the best evidence available, in consultation with the patient, to decide upon the option which suits that patient best' (Muir Gray 1997a, p. 9).

'Evidence-based medicine requires you to … read the right papers at the right time and then to alter your behaviour (and, what is often more difficult, the behaviour of other people) in the light of what you have found.' (Greenhalgh 2001, p. 2).

AN INTER-DISCIPLINARY APPROACH TO EVIDENCE-BASED PRACTICE

Evidence-based practice initially developed using a uniprofessional model within medicine. In subsequent years, with the development of clinical governance for all professions, other groups in health and social care adapted this model to suit their practice. Originally, this remained predominantly confined to single professional groups but more recently, policy has emphasised inter-disciplinary and generic models. Similarly, stakeholders (that is managers, commissioners, service users, educators and researchers) are interested in the effectiveness of the entire team rather than the single intervention of one profession. In most cases an intervention does not occur in isolation from other treatments and from the patient's or user's point of view it is the outcome of the entire experience that is important. Thus evidence-based practice is moving from a model where individual professions evaluate their own interventions to one where teams consider the effect of the entire treatment process. However, single professional interventions are still important. As a patient visiting a physiotherapist for back pain you want to know that the interventions that are used work, or at the very least, do not do any harm. Similarly, users of a community mental health team want to know that the kind of care offered has a better, or at least as good an outcome as that provided using other models of care.

Whether you look for evidence to support a single intervention by one profession or whether you look at the effectiveness of the whole package of care largely depends on the nature of your work. However, evaluating outcomes of a single intervention is difficult as it is virtually impossible to exclude the potential effects of the other interventions occurring at the same time. It is also potentially meaningless as service users do not usually experience their care as a series of separate interventions. If current trends in the delivery of health and social care continue then the following discussions will increasingly relate to the interventions offered by the entire team and all AHPs, at whatever level, will have a responsibility to ensure their practice is evidence-based.

So what do you have to do to be an evidence-based practitioner? Most authors agree that evidence-based practice consists of five stages:

1. Asking the right question.
2. Finding and accessing the evidence.
3. Critically evaluating the evidence.
4. Implementing changes based on the evidence.
5. Evaluating and monitoring the effect of these changes.

Asking the right question

For a novice practitioner working out the right question to ask is probably the most difficult stage and the part that is least considered. Although it may sometimes seem that the questions we need to ask are relatively straightforward, Law (2002) contends that in order to be able to ask the right kind of questions you first need to develop skills necessary for reflective practice. Additionally, Dawes (1999a) argues that to be a good professional you need to develop a questioning attitude to your work. This is supported by Muir Gray (1997b) who suggests we must consider such questions as: Are the interventions that you are using proven to be effective? Are you carrying them out in the right way and are they occurring at the right time?

One of the most common difficulties novice practitioners have when starting to formulate questions is that they are too broad and hence are unlikely to produce any useful information. For example occupational therapists often advise people with rheumatoid arthritis on techniques designed to protect joints and preserve function, but what is the evidence to support the use of these techniques? As an initial question this in itself may be reasonable, but is still rather broad. You may not be certain that people follow the joint protection techniques that they have been shown, so a more specific question might be 'Do people with rheumatoid arthritis who have been instructed in joint preservation techniques have improved function in their hands after 5 years compared to people who have not had intervention?' Or 'Do people use joint-protection techniques after being instructed?' If you want to be sure that you are doing things in the right way your question might be 'What are joint protection techniques and are some more effective than others?' To find out if you are doing things at the right time the question might be 'Is it better to introduce joint protection techniques as soon as possible after diagnosis?' You may also want to know about the cost effectiveness of your intervention so you may ask 'Does instruction in joint protection techniques reduce the need for joint replacement surgery?'

To summarise then, first in order to ensure that you are asking the right question you need to define your problem clearly (if there is no problem there is no question); second narrow down the problem to a question, and third define the question into something simple that can be answered. Questions may be about cause and effect, can consider associations between things, can summarise the results of other information and can describe things.

Levels of evidence

Once you have worked out what you want to know the second step is to evaluate the evidence. In order to do that you need to know what constitutes 'evidence.' Although there are many ways of categorising and describing different

Table 9.1

Level	Type of evidence
1	Strong evidence from at least one published systematic review of multiple, well-designed randomised controlled trials
2	Strong evidence from at least one published properly designed randomised controlled trial of appropriate size and in an appropriate clinical setting
3	Evidence from well-designed trials without randomisation, single group, pre, post-cohort, time series or matched case-controlled studies
4	Evidence from well-designed non-experimental studies from more than one centre or research group
5	Opinions of respected authorities based on clinical evidence, descriptive studies or reports of expert consensus committees

types of evidence, I have based this discussion on the 'levels of evidence' (see Table 9.1) suggested by a print and internet journal called *Bandolier*. This publication uses evidence-based medicine techniques to provide advice about particular treatments or diseases for healthcare professionals and consumers (*Bandolier* 1994, accessed 19/11/2003).

Systematic reviews

A systematic review is an overview of primary research in a particular area that has been carried out using a specific and reproducible methodology. It starts with a clearly formulated question and involves a defined and extensive review of the literature, a critical and objective evaluation of all of the evidence and an appraisal based on pre-defined criteria. This rigour in methods differentiates it from general reviews published in professional journals and the kind of reviews that you might carry out for an undergraduate essay. It is tempting to consider carrying out a systematic review as an alternative to primary research, thinking that this might be more straightforward. However, the opposite is true as you need advanced skills of critical analysis and a thorough understanding of research methods often only gained at doctoral or post-doctoral level. You may also hear the term 'meta-analyses' alongside systematic reviews. A meta-analysis is 'the statistical synthesis of the numerical results of several trials which all address the same question' (Greenhalgh 2001, p. 127). It is mostly carried out by or with the help of statisticians with an interest and expertise in these kinds of analyses.

When looking for evidence to answer your questions, the best thing that you can hope for is that someone has already carried out and published a good and recent systematic review that will answer some aspects of your question. Good quality systematic reviews are published in most academic journals; however a good starting point is the Cochrane database of systematic reviews. The Cochrane Centre was set up to facilitate systematic reviews of randomised controlled trials nationally and internationally and the database contains reviews conducted by the Cochrane Centre itself and other researchers.

Randomised controlled trials and experimental research

In clinically based experimental research you are trying to measure the effect of your intervention (the independent variable) on a previously defined factor (the dependent variable). The most usual way of doing this is a randomised controlled trial, although there are other methods.

Randomised controlled trials are one of the most highly rated sources of clinical evidence in health or social care. In a randomised controlled trial participants are randomly assigned to a treatment group or a control group so that the effect of the intervention can be studied. Both groups are evaluated at the beginning and end of the intervention using a predetermined set of measures. It is the randomisation of participants to the two groups that is important as the premise of these studies is that because participants are assigned randomly the two groups are considered to be broadly the same and hence any differences in the results of the groups are due to the intervention. There can be ethical issues concerned with denying the intervention to the control group, although if you don't know whether the intervention works it is not ethical to use it anyway.

Randomised controlled trials can be challenging to design and costly to administer but provide powerful evidence. Smith et al. (accessed 17/11/03) reviewed a number of studies looking at the effectiveness of acupuncture in pain relief for people who have had a stroke and present a good discussion on the difficulties with randomised controlled trials. (This paper is in the *Bandolier* journal and can be accessed online.)

Quasi-experimental research

Batavia (2001) defines quasi-experimental research as being similar to experimental research (you are still testing the effect of the independent variable on the dependent variable) but either it has not been possible to randomise participants to a control and intervention group or there is no comparison group. Royeen (1997) argues that as randomisation is virtually impossible in clinical settings most clinically based research tends to be quasi-experimental in design. There are many different types of studies that fall into this category, but the important thing is that the study has been well-designed. Experimental and quasi-experimental designs are highly controlled in relation to the sample chosen, the measures used, data collection and data analysis.

Within subject or repeated measures designs are an example of quasi-experimental studies. They are often used to compare two or more different treatments. The participants are measured at the start and then given treatments in various orders or combinations. There is no control group or randomisation but the way or order in which the interventions are applied is strictly controlled. Measures are taken at each stage and eventually all participants receive all interventions. Another example is single subject studies, where research on a single participant or a number of participants is carried out using an experimental design. Typically the participant is assessed prior to intervention to obtain a baseline measure, the intervention is carried out, and the participant is reassessed. There are no control groups.

Descriptive research

A lot of research carried out by allied health and social care professionals falls into the category of descriptive research. Although not as highly rated as experimental and quasi-experimental research, descriptive research provides answers to some pertinent questions in our field. Descriptive research uses both quantitative and qualitative methodologies and can be correlational, survey research or clinical description (Royeen 1997).

Correlation studies aim to describe and measure the relationship between things (such as 'mood' and 'memory' or 'cardiovascular fitness' and 'well-being'). Data are collected on a number of variables and a series of statistical analyses are carried out to explore the associations between them. Correlational research looks at relationships between things but does not look at cause and effect.

Survey research is usually quantitative in design and aims to gain information about or from a large group of people by systematically surveying a smaller but representative group. Surveys often use questionnaires as a data collection tool, but can also use other methods such as face-to-face interviews, telephone interviews and internet surveying.

Clinical studies describe clinical things, such as the numbers of people diagnosed with a particular disease, or may be a description of an interesting or unusual case (case reports). Although this type of study is not ranked high in the evidence tree, Greenhalgh (2001) argues that case reports are very useful as they are often easily understandable, can be written up rapidly and bring information that is potentially important quickly into the public arena.

Qualitative studies are usually carried out to answer the questions that seek to understand people's experience, attitudes or beliefs and mostly aim to generate rich and meaningful data but do not, and in most cases cannot, generalise these results beyond the study group. Although qualitative studies are not rated as highly as experimental designs they are increasingly gaining in importance because they answer questions that enable us to understand the patients' or clients' experiences, and this is what service users repeatedly say they want from health and social care professionals. Evidence-based practice requires us to use the available evidence to work with service users to agree on the right intervention and this is only possible if you have some understanding of their experiences. There are many different paradigms, methods and designs for qualitative studies. Three common design types are ethnography, phenomenology and grounded theory. Grbich (1999), Holloway (1997) and Denzin and Lincoln (1994) are good resources for a more detailed discussion on qualitative methods and designs.

Finding and accessing the evidence

Having considered what constitutes evidence the next task is finding it. The growth of the internet and online search facilities has made this task much easier and made a great deal of material accessible. Even if you do not have access to an academic library or your own computer you can access the internet from most public libraries. That is not to say that the internet is the best source or should be your only source, but judicious use can certainly point you in the right direction for further searching.

The Cochrane Collaboration Handbook (Clarke and Oxman 2003) recommends the following strategies for carrying out an effective review. Start first with a computer search using electronic databases. The databases you choose to search will be guided by your question, but those most commonly used are ASSIA (Applied Social Sciences Indexes and Abstracts); MEDLINE (the online version of Index Medicus); EMBASE (the database of Excerpta Medica; this has broader European coverage than Medline); CINAHL (Cumulative Index to Nursing and Allied Health Literature); PSYCINFO (Database from the American Psychological Society); and AMED (Allied and Alternative Medicine Database). Snowball (1999) provides a detailed list of resources including databases, online and print journals. However, this information goes out of date quickly and should always be checked with an informed librarian or on the National electronic Library for Health (NeHL). This is still in its infancy but provides an online library service for healthcare workers and the general public. It has specialist portals for various professions and provides links to electronic databases and other sources of evidence. It is a good starting point for any search on questions about health and healthcare.

Carrying out an online database search is a skilled task and if you haven't done it before the best thing is to get a more experienced researcher or librarian to show you. The key is to enter the words into the search in the right combination so that you get as good a coverage as possible but are selective enough in order that you don't end up with thousands of citations. Snowball (1999) calls this the trade-off between comprehensiveness and selectivity. If your online search produces no citations then unless you have picked a topic that no one else has ever thought about, the chances are you are doing it incorrectly. It may be that no one else has asked your specific question, but it is highly unlikely that no one else has been interested in a similar topic but with a different client group, or a slightly different topic but asking similar questions. Finally, it is imperative to search more than one database to ensure that you have got as broad a coverage as possible.

It is often necessary to follow up a computer search by hand searching or citation tracking. This involves looking through the indexes and copies of any key journals to search out relevant papers. You may need to do this because not all studies or journals are listed in electronic databases and even if they are, they may not be written in a way that makes them easily picked up by a keyword search.

Hopefully your computer search will have highlighted a number of relevant papers. Abstracts are often available online and by reading them you can get an indication as to whether the paper is relevant. However, if the paper looks relevant from the abstract always get a full copy. In addition, when following up citations from other papers, you should try to obtain a copy of the original source and not rely on someone else's interpretation of the information.

This strategy refers to published peer reviewed journal articles, but there is a lot of evidence that does not fall into this category. Because some of it may not be rigorously peer reviewed you must use it cautiously; however it is still important and can provide the most recent information and information that is relevant at a local level.

Many researchers choose to present their current research at conferences prior to full publication, so searching conference proceedings and abstracts may find the most recent research in your field. Similarly, a lot of research that is carried out for higher degrees remains unpublished but can be accessed through theses collections and university libraries. Evaluations, service reviews and small research projects may be commissioned by local services and special interest groups. These may be written up as reports for local distribution or reported on an organisation's web pages. Voluntary organisations and pressure groups will often be aware of ongoing research relevant to their field and report it on their web pages or in newsletters. Another way of getting in touch with experts in your field and keeping up with current debate is via internet discussion groups. Many professions have their own groups on a variety of topics and links to them can be found from the web pages of professional associations.

Although the internet has revolutionised our ability to access details of the most recent advances it has also created a problem as information accessed online can be of varying quality. The internet should never be your only or primary source of evidence and material obtained in this way needs to be critically reviewed and if possible supported by published peer-reviewed studies.

Critically evaluating the evidence

Once you have identified the question and tracked down all the available evidence the next stage is to formulate a critique. This part of becoming an evidence-based practitioner presents one of the biggest challenges to new practitioners, as it requires a high level of skill usually developed at postgraduate level. There are many standard formats available that will help you to adopt a scientific approach to critical appraisal; however there are some points to consider before beginning.

First, you must actually read the paper or study thoroughly. Dawes (1999b) makes the point that in many cases people begin a critical review without having spent enough time reading the paper in the first place.

Second, you need to begin your review from a neutral position and, at this point, put your own ideas and thoughts to one side. For example, you may believe passionately that cognitive–behavioural therapy is the best intervention for people with anxiety, but when you find a study that suggests that it offers no lasting benefits over and above other interventions, you must approach it the same way as you would a study that concludes that it has positive benefits. This may sound like stating the obvious, but developing this neutral starting point is one of the hardest parts of the process and requires the development of personal skills such as self-awareness and reflexivity in order for you to truly master this aspect. It is also important to remember that critiquing something doesn't mean just being negative but it is an analysis and judgement of a piece of work based on its merit. Your final conclusions may ultimately be positive.

There are four things you need to consider when reviewing an evidence-based paper. These concern the research question, design, analysis and interpretation. The first point to consider is have they asked the right question? Previously we saw that working out what you want to find out is one of the most difficult parts of evidence-based practice. In a good paper the research question and aims of the research will be clearly stated and supported by the literature. The most common things that are wrong with research questions is that they do not ask anything worth asking (there is no problem), they are not adequately justified in relation to previous research or they are too general.

Once the question is clear you need to consider the adequacy of the research design. There are two main aspects to consider. First, is the type of design appropriate for the research question and second, has the study been designed well enough to answer the research question? It is the nature of the research question that determines the design and not the other way round. A common mistake that those new to research often make is to decide on a design (such as a survey) before defining the problem. Batavia (2001, p. 37) provides an excellent flow diagram to show how types of questions fit with different research designs.

Key points

- Questions concerning cause and effect are usually experimental or quasi-experimental.
- Questions considering the association or relationships between things use correlational designs.
- Questions wanting to describe things use descriptive methods, which can be qualitative or quantitative.

The second part to assessing design is whether the study has been designed well enough to answer the research question. In order to evaluate a paper effectively you need an understanding of all of the research designs described earlier in this chapter. This is quite a daunting task for a novice practitioner, but fortunately there are several guides already available to assist you in doing this. The most straightforward are those from Law et al. (1998), which can be downloaded directly from the McMaster's University website. They provide separate guidelines for qualitative and quantitative studies.

If the study appears to be well-designed the next thing to consider is whether the data has been analysed adequately. This is the point at which many people feel panic at the thought of having to understand complex statistical analyses. This fear is mostly unfounded, as you do not necessarily need to understand the mathematical workings for most straightforward statistics but you should consider whether the right kind of statistical test has been used and whether the procedure has been clearly documented. Statistics are best learnt by practising them yourself on your own data and although there are several good books on statistical analyses most people find it hard to learn in this way. If the statistics in the paper are too much for you, do what many experienced researchers do and ask a statistician. When reviewing data analysis in qualitative studies the principles are similar in that you need to ask whether the methods of data analysis have been clearly described, were the appropriate methods chosen and do the results clearly emerge from the data.

The final aspect to consider is whether the results have been interpreted correctly. Results of research are usually presented tentatively as it is impossible to design a perfect piece of research and so conclusions are always open to some challenge. Important points to consider are whether the conclusions of the study are reasonable, can the results be generalised and what are the implications for practice. Research claiming to have found something remarkable very rarely has.

Communicating the evidence

As discussed earlier in this chapter, being an evidence-based practitioner is more than being aware of the evidence, but is a way of integrating the results of the evidence with your own clinical reasoning and the user/patient/clients' wishes. For this to be successful, evidence must be disseminated. Most people think of publication in a professional journal as the most important way of communicating research evidence. Indeed the importance of publication to ensure research funding and secure academic jobs has never been stronger. However, the emphasis on this type of academic writing has perhaps been to the detriment of other methods, which may, in fact, achieve a greater coverage. The important things to think about are who do I want to read this information and what is the aim?

To be an evidence-based practitioner you need to first be able to communicate details of the evidence with your patients and clients. In a clinical setting verbal explanations are essential, but people often find it difficult to remember or take in information after a consultation. (All of us have had the experience of realising once we have left the doctor's surgery that we have forgotten what was said.) Verbal explanations can be followed up by written material and you should be prepared to repeat information several times. It is important to strike a balance when communicating to avoid being patronising, but keeping explanations in non-technical or 'lay' terms. Exactly how you communicate information will also depend on the needs of your patients and clients and take into account any communication problems that they might have.

If the aim of communicating the results of your evidence is to change local practice and to influence local stakeholders with regard to your service then a simple written report for local dissemination may be most effective. Follow local guidelines with regard to the format and style of the report. Written reports of this type are likely to be more effective when combined with a short presentation as this ensures that people read the report and gives an opportunity for discussion.

If you wish to influence profession-specific practice, communicating within a professional group is likely to be most effective and you have many options. If your topic is related to a specialist area of practice, professional sub-groups or specialist sections will enable you to access key people in that field. This can be via meetings, newsletters, conferences or in some cases, a specialist journal. If the topic is of general professional interest, a poster or paper at a professional conference or publication in a professional journal is more effective. If your topic is something of international interest publication in an international journal should be considered. International journals vary in quality but those that are peer reviewed generally have a higher 'impact factor' than national publications. The impact factor of a journal is an indication of its quality based on the frequency with which the journal's articles are cited in other scientific publications.

Earlier on in the chapter we considered the fact that, increasingly, the search for evidence will be an inter-professional collaboration. This research is better communicated with the wider professional audience, at a local, national and international level. Again this may be via inter-professional papers, posters or reports.

Generally, the results of health and social care research are often poorly communicated to the wider public. This is in contrast to medical research which is widely reported in newspapers and on the television. Even if your project is not worthy of national press coverage, special interest groups, lobby groups and voluntary organisations may be interested. A journal with a high impact factor will often have far fewer readers than a regular publication by a charity or national special interest group such as the Stroke Association.

Implementing changes based on evidence

The final two stages of becoming an evidence-based practitioner involve implementing changes based on evidence and evaluating the effect of these changes. Although communicating evidence is relatively straightforward once you have decided what you want to communicate and to whom, implementing any change is more difficult and changes that are system wide are even more difficult to effect at a novice-practitioner level. Change can occur on many levels from the national and strategic level, to the local and individual level (Davies 1999). In the early stages of your career it is most likely that you will be involved at the local and individual level, which means implementing changes to your own practice and within the team or service in which you work.

The easiest changes to carry out are those to your own practice and may come about after a detailed search of the literature, reflecting on your current practice and discussion in supervision. They might include changing your approach to a particular client or client group, or modifying the way you carry out an intervention. You may also need to consider taking part in further or advanced training to update your skills. Any change must be supported by current evidence, should only be effected with the support of your supervisor and should be documented and evaluated.

Changes may also be carried out at the service level and although they are usually initiated by senior members of the team, it is often students or new practitioners that have the most current access to the latest evidence. A team that encourages critical and open reflection on current practice through regular meetings, audit, journal clubs and supervision is likely to be more open to considering changes in practice. Evidence shows that good leadership and management is also essential in order to initiate change.

Other barriers to change highlighted by professionals themselves are lack of evidence, lack of skills, lack of time, lack of resources, difficulty accessing information and lack of support. It is also difficult to implement change if people feel it will make their current job more difficult or will not offer any clear benefits over current practice.

Evaluating and monitoring changes

If you are a reflective practitioner then evaluating and monitoring changes at an individual level will be an implicit part of your practice. Initially this may be through a reflective diary, supervision and peer feedback, but may lead to a more formal evaluation. For example, after researching the evidence and undertaking further training you may adapt an aspect of your intervention. You then need to evaluate the effect that these changes have made. Have patient outcomes changed, are you carrying out the techniques in the correct way, does it take longer than the previous methods and importantly are these methods still up to date? The process for monitoring and evaluating change at a service level is audit, and this is explained elsewhere in this book.

SUMMARY

To summarise the key points of this chapter, evidence-based practice is now part and parcel of modern-day health and social care and all practitioners need to be able to demonstrate competence in this field. It is not only about keeping up with the latest research evidence, but being able to evaluate it, reflect on it and integrate it into your own clinical practice. To be an evidence-based practitioner you require skills of critical appraisal, clinical expertise and self-reflection and you must apply these creatively and scientifically in partnership with your clients or patients.

Key points

■ Evidence-based practice means being familiar with the most recent evidence and using that knowledge, together with clinical judgement, to work with the patient or client.
■ To be an evidence-based practitioner you need to be a reflective practitioner and develop your skills of critical analysis.

Useful websites

http://www.york.ac.uk/inst/crd/
The University of York NHS Centre for reviews and dissemination – and the Database of Abstracts and Reviews of Effects (DARE)

http://www.nelh.nhs.uk/
National electronic Library for Health and Social Care

http://www.nice.org.uk/
National Centre for Clinical Excellence systematic appraisal of health interventions

http://cebmh.warne.ox.ac.uk/cebmh/
Evidence-based practice in mental health

http://www.jr2.ox.ac.uk/bandolier/index.html
Bandolier – internet journal

http://www.cochrane.org/index0.htm
The Cochrane Collaboration

http://www.kingsfund.org.uk/
The Kings Fund

http://www.elsc.org.uk/
Electronic library for social care

http://www.hda-online.org.uk/evidence/
Evidence base for public health

http://www.otseeker.com/
A database that contains abstracts of systematic reviews and randomised controlled trials relevant to occupational therapy

http://www.pedro.fhs.usyd.edu.au/
The Physiotherapy Evidence Database

REFERENCES

Bandolier 1994 *Assessment criteria; type and strength of evidence.*
   Online. Available:
   http://www.jr2.ox.ac.uk/bandolier/band6/b6-5.html
   19 Nov 2003.

Batavia M 2001 *Clinical research for health professionals.* Butterworth Heinemann, Boston.

Clarke M, Oxman AD (eds) 2003 *Locating and selecting studies for reviews.* Cochrane
   Reviewers' Handbook 4.2.0 (updated March 2003); Section 5.
   Online. Available:
   http://www.cochrane.dk/cochrane/handbook/handbook.htm
   03 Nov 2003.

Davies P 1999 Introducing change. In: Dawes M, Davies PT, Gray AM et al. (eds) *Evidence-
   based practice: a primer for healthcare professionals.* Churchill Livingstone, Edinburgh,
   pp. 203–218.

Dawes M 1999a Formulating a question. In: Dawes M, Davies PT, Gray AM et al. (eds)
   Evidence-based practice: a primer for healthcare professionals. Churchill Livingstone,
   Edinburgh, pp. 9–13.

Dawes M 1999b Introduction to critical appraisal. In: Dawes M, Davies PT, Gray AM et al.
   (eds) *Evidence-based practice: a primer for healthcare professionals.* Churchill Livingstone,
   Edinburgh, pp. 47–48.

Denzin NK, Lincoln YS (eds) 1994 *Handbook of qualitative research.* Sage, Thousand Oaks.

Greenhalgh T 2001 *How to read a paper – the basics of evidence-based medicine.* BMJ Books,
   London.

Grbich C 1999 *Qualitative research in health.* Sage, London.

Holloway I 1997 *Basic concepts for qualitative research.* Blackwell Science, Oxford.

Law M 2002 *Evidence-based rehabilitation: a guide to practice.* Slack, Thorofare.

Law M, Stewart D, Letts L, Pollark M, Bosch J, Westmorland M 1998 *Guidelines for critical
   review form – qualitative studies.*
   Online. Available:
   http://www-fhs.mcmaster.ca/rehab/ebp/pdf/qualguidelines.pdf
   17 November 2003.

Muir Gray JA 1997a Evidence-based healthcare. In: *Evidence-based healthcare: how to make
   health policy and management decisions.* Churchill Livingstone, Edinburgh, pp.1–16.

Muir Gray JA 1997b Doing the right things right. In: *Evidence-based healthcare: how to make
   health policy and management decisions.* Churchill Livingstone, Edinburgh, pp. 17–27.

Royeen CB 1997 *A research primer in occupational and physical therapy.* American Occupational
   Therapy Association, Bethesda, MD.

Sackett DL, Rosenberg WM, Gray JA, Haynes RB, Richardson WS 1996 Evidence-based medicine: what it is and what it isn't. *British Medical Journal* 312(7023): 71–72.

Smith L, Moore O, McQuay H, Moore A 2003 *Assessing the evidence of effectiveness of acupuncture for stroke rehabilitation: stepped assessment of likelihood of bias.*
   Online. Available:
   http://www.jr2.ox.ac.uk/bandolier/booth/alternat/ACstroke.html
   11 March 2003.

Snowball R 1999 Finding the evidence: An information skills approach. In: Dawes M, Davies
   PT, Gray AM et al (eds) *Evidence-based practice: a primer for healthcare professionals.*
   Churchill Livingstone, Edinburgh, pp. 15–46.

Audit in allied health professional practice

Robin Sasaru, Yvette Sheward and
Soma Sasaru

LEARNING OUTCOMES

The learning outcomes that will be addressed in this chapter are to:
- Define what clinical audit is.
- Describe the audit cycle.
- Select criteria for clinical audit.
- Measure performance and compare with criteria.
- Propose improvements based on audit data.

INTRODUCTION

Looking to 'do a clinical audit'? Not sure where to start? Not sure what clinical audit is? Maybe you have heard a lot about clinical audit, and often viewpoints on the definition of clinical audit differ. With this chapter, hopefully you will see how audit can be used to best effect to make improvements in the quality of your care.

Reflective questions:

Key questions to think about as you read this chapter are:

- *How would you define clinical audit?*
- *Where does the audit cycle start?*
- *What should you consider before you start an audit project?*

WHAT IS CLINICAL AUDIT?

Clinical audit has been redefined on and off, over the last 15 years, in the light of new understanding and direction. Originally, medical audit (as it was called) was aimed at 'peer reviewing' the quality of medical care. During the 1990s the emphasis of clinical audit for all healthcare professionals came to the fore, causing many medical audit departments to purchase new 'clinical audit' signage for their front doors. Clinical audit has more recently been re-aligned towards multidisciplinary, multi-professional, multi-agency, (and even multi-media) working. The advent of clinical governance has enabled clinical audit to be seen as one of several key pillars supporting quality improvement in the National Health Service (NHS).

The most recent, and perhaps most definitive definition of clinical audit is as follows:

> *Clinical audit is a quality improvement process that seeks to improve patient care and outcomes through systematic review of care against explicit criteria and the implementation of change. Aspects of the structure, processes, and outcomes of care are selected and systematically evaluated against explicit criteria. Where indicated, changes are implemented at an individual, team, or service level and further monitoring is used to confirm improvement in healthcare delivery.*

(National Institute of Clinical Excellence [NICE] 2002)

If you like, clinical audit looks at the following in a thorough, methodical way:

- Measuring the quality of care given to patients ('current practice').
- Comparing this measure with what care should be given ('best practice').
- Making changes to improve the quality of care.
- Confirming that those changes have resulted in improvement.

Clinical audit has some hallmarks that distinguish it from other activities:

- Quality improvement.
- Systematic review.
- Explicit criteria.
- Continuing process.

Quality improvement (of patient care and outcomes) is the prime reason for conducting clinical audit. From this we see that clinical audit projects are not simply reports of activity or throughput, and are not done simply 'to see what is going on' in an area. As all improvement requires change, the implementation of change is included as a part of the process of audit.

Clinical audit is also characterised by systematic review. 'Systematic' can be defined as 'methodical' or 'orderly', so good audit projects should provide evidence of a well thought out, step-by-step approach to quality improvement. This approach can be far more effective than an intuitive approach. It follows that if we are to be systematic in the way we conduct audit, we should also be systematic in the way we choose topics for clinical audit.

Explicit criteria form another hallmark of all clinical audit, one that sets audit apart from most other quality improvement processes. These criteria are obtained by using the principles of clinical effectiveness (doing the right thing to the right person at the right time). Explicit criteria provide the 'golden line' of excellent quality care that, ideally, all patients should receive. Also, because these criteria are measurable, they can enable you to make reliable, repeatable comparisons between the 'golden line' and the actual care that takes place.

Further monitoring is also included in the audit cycle, as all clinical audit projects should be regarded as continuous. Not all change is improvement – so having a step to confirm that the changes you make actually result in better patient care is very useful.

AUDIT IS INTEGRAL TO HEALTHCARE

The NHS is increasingly coming under internal and external scrutiny. Information from clinical audit projects is therefore useful to help provide answers for all those examining NHS organisations.

Clinical audit is one of the major components of clinical governance (see Chapter 8). Clinical governance asks for a well-conducted clinical audit programme, linked in to all the other aspects of its domain:

- Clinical audit.
- Clinical effectiveness.
- Staffing and staff management.
- Patient and public involvement.
- Risk management.
- Education and development.
- Use of information.

RESEARCH VS AUDIT

Research

Research aims to increase the sum of academic knowledge by establishing facts that can be generalised to a population. Research could ask 'what is the best thing to do?' or 'what is the best way to do something?'

Quantitative research, for example, in the form of randomised controlled trials is a type of research favoured by some practitioners in health. These types of studies are often designed to answer whether a particular treatment or intervention is more effective than a 'control group', which may receive a different intervention, no intervention, or a placebo. Research activities include all forms of experimental trial and other forms of enquiry (see Chapter 9).

Research in the NHS requires ethical approval in all instances, and needs to be registered with the appropriate research and development groups within your Trust.

Clinical audit

Clinical audit asks 'how does the care that we provide compare with established standards for best practice?' Clinical audit does not increase the sum of human knowledge as research does, and it does not provide facts that can be generalised to a population.

Figure 10.1
Audit cycle – audit, a continuous process, can be best described as a cycle or spiral.

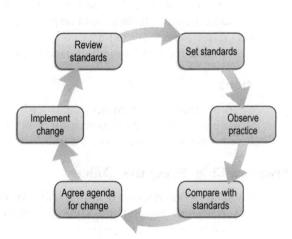

Although methodology is shared with audit (rigorous, systematic), the comparison made is always standard vs. practice, with no control group. Audit usually does not require ethical approval (but should always be registered with your organisation's clinical audit/governance structure). For details of the audit cycle see Figure 10.1.

PREPARING FOR AUDIT

The foundation of any good audit project is proper preparation. Without it, your audit will not deliver improvements in healthcare. What is required for this good foundation?

Accountabilities and structures

Your NHS organisation has a statutory duty of quality – and will have organisational structures in place to make assurances regarding the quality of care to the Trust Board. Clinical audit is normally part of this structure.

Roles and responsibilities

In addition to your own professional responsibility to provide high-quality care, there will be key people within your organisation who have a responsibility for ensuring and improving quality. Usually, your particular service area will have a lead person responsible for some or all aspects of clinical governance, including clinical audit.

Contacting your organisation's lead for clinical audit might help you gather some ideas on how best to go forward with an audit activity in your department.

Patients/service users

The main purpose of clinical audit is to improve patient care and outcomes, so audit should be compatible with patient, public and carer involvement. There are many bodies and committees related to the NHS that can help you to obtain this type of input. As the viewpoint and experience of the patient is very different from that of the health professional, involving them can pay dividends in helping to understand what actually happens in your service, and how to make it better. Patients are usually experts in their health problem and the care of it – so all within the audit team should respect their views as such. The Patient Advice and Liaison Service (PALS) have co-ordinators or support workers that you can consult to action involvement of patients and the public in your audit project.

Partner organisations

When a clinical audit project deals with the interface or handover of care between more than one organisation or department, it is important to have all these interests represented on the audit team.

Managers/Directors/Chief Executive Officer

As well as having relevant frontline staff involved in the audit, you must get your organisation to 'sign-off' the audit. The higher the level of authorisation and commitment to your project, the more likely you are going to improve practice as a result. It is therefore helpful to get your director or head of service to support your audit project. Get them (as well as your immediate line manager) to agree to provide protected time to complete the audit.

AUDIT AND CLINICAL GOVERNANCE

Clinical audit is seen as a key part of the clinical governance arrangements within all NHS trusts. Audit is best conducted as part of a structured and prioritised programme.

Accessing your organisation's clinical governance structure

Clinical governance is a framework through which NHS organisations are responsible and accountable for continuously improving the quality of their services as well as safeguarding high standards of care and creating an environment in which excellence in clinical care can flourish (Department of Health [DoH] 1998).

What does this mean? Well, all NHS organisations must demonstrate that the quality of care they provide is continually improving. To do this they must set up a culture of improvement; clinical staff should be able to participate in making changes to the way services are delivered. In addition to setting up this culture, NHS organisations must structure the way improvements are made. Usually this is done by setting up committees, groups, or teams with responsibilities related to clinical governance. In every trust clinical audit is considered by one or more committees somewhere along the line. Remember that ensuring organisational commitment to audit provides a sound basis for making changes that result from your audit project.

Resources (including funding) for clinical audit in your trust

Many NHS trusts have resources dedicated to clinical audit. Usually this support is in the form of one or more clinical audit facilitators. Clinical audit facilitators are experienced staff with knowledge of the audit cycle, and they can provide much practical help with your audit project.

Because audit projects usually require a commitment of your time, it is vital to check with your supervisor/line manager that you can have the time to do the audit. Some people feel that, because the audit project is important to them, they are happy to do it 'in their own time'. Consider though, if your manager is unwilling to give you time to complete the audit project, might they also be unwilling to make changes to the service as a result of your project? If the topic in question is a priority to the service, then there should be agreement to give you the time to do the work.

Registration and monitoring of audit activities

Audit activity within an NHS organisation should be registered at some level. Usually your clinical audit department will be able to tell you how to go about registering an audit project within your organisation. This is an important part of organisational protocol; do not start a project without registering it! Registration of audit projects is valuable because:

■ NHS organisations must produce an annual clinical audit report, for discussion at board level. Registration of audit projects helps the staff concerned to quickly collect data on the audit projects that have been completed over the specified year.
■ Registration of audit projects helps to avoid duplication and wasted effort.

Project teams for clinical audit

To produce a successful audit, projects need to involve key individuals, those who have the right skills and knowledge in the service area being reviewed. This means that in addition to clinicians and audit staff, it is also important to include all other relevant staff involved in the delivery of care and not purely those with clinical experience. This could for example include administrative or other support staff. To make improvements in the quality of care it is necessary to have an understanding of all processes and systems used within the service and this can only be achieved by involving those who work there. To enable this, all team members should have an understanding of the aims and objectives of the audit and also what is expected of the project team.

SELECTING TOPICS

Since one of the hallmarks of clinical audit is a systematic approach, it follows that audit topics should also be decided on in a systematic way. NICE (2002) for example, suggest that clinical audit is best carried out within a structured programme and supported by a strong team approach with participation by all staff and effective leadership.

Topics and prioritisation

Resources in the NHS are finite and limited. For this reason, topics for clinical audit must be selected with careful thought and planning. Resist the desire to audit your favourite subject or condition without thinking about other priorities. When considering which topic to audit, some useful questions to ask are:

■ What is associated with high risk/volume/cost to staff or patients/service users?
■ Is there evidence of a serious quality problem? (Existing data may tell you this.)
■ Is there high quality clinical evidence to base practice standards on?
■ Is there a strong likelihood that this audit will result in changes (improvements)?
■ Is there any national audit work going on in this area?
■ Are there any national policies that relate to this area?
■ Is the topic a priority for my organisation?

The more questions you can answer 'yes' to, the more likely your audit topic will be of high priority to the organisation. A significant incident or complaint can also give you ideas about topics to audit. Basing audit topics around complaints or incidents in this manner is highly beneficial, as it can help to prevent such things happening again.

DEVELOPING STANDARDS AND SELECTING CRITERIA

The main thrust of a clinical audit report is to compare patient care and outcomes with agreed standards for the service, by using explicit criteria. It is important then to know:

- What are standards and criteria?
- How are standards set and how are criteria selected?

Selecting criteria

In order to select the best criteria it is important to be clear about what they are. Criteria have been defined for some time, clearly linking to their usefulness in audit. According to Irvine and Irvine (1991), they are a measurable item of healthcare that both describes quality and can be used to assess it. Similarly, the Institute of Medicine (1992), suggests that criteria are systematically developed statements that can be used to assess not only the appropriateness of specific healthcare decisions but also services and outcomes. From these definitions you can see that criteria used in clinical audit are really measures. Criteria measure the quality of healthcare.

For this to be true, people engaged in audit need to select the right measures! The criteria used need to be proportional to the aspect of quality being looked at. For instance, if you wanted to check the speed of your car as you are driving, you would look at the readout on your speedometer. Looking at the time would not tell you what speed you are travelling at – because it is the wrong measure for what you need to know. There are three main types of criteria, or measures, used in clinical audit:

- *Structure* – what you need – the fuel gauge.
- *Process* – what you do – the rev counter.
- *Outcome* – what you expect – the speedometer.

Structure criteria measure the available resources and their organisation, such as number of staff, provision of equipment, physical space, etc. This is just like a fuel gauge on a car, which measures how much fuel resource you have available. Structure criteria will not tell you whether you are using these resources wisely or if you are getting the right patient care outcomes. However, if the structure is not right, then auditing process or outcome may not result in major improvements.

Process criteria measure the action taken (the doing) by a healthcare team, such as communication, assessment, investigation, intervention, evaluation, documentation, etc. This is just like a rev counter, which measures what the engine is doing. Process criteria can be of great value in 'fine-tuning' the process and increase its efficiency. Auditing process criteria are only valuable if you have a good understanding of the process. Generally, auditing using process criteria is not valuable if you know that your structure is not up to scratch. (No point fretting why the rev counter fails to move if you know you are out of fuel.)

Outcome criteria measure the actual response to the intervention, such as the reported health status, level of knowledge, etc. This is like the speedometer on a car, which measures the actual speed you are travelling at. Outcome criteria, while useful, must be treated with caution, as outcomes are dependent on more than just the process of care. Factors external to the process, such as case mix, may need to be accounted for. (If your car is stuck in the mud, you can rev the engine all you like and be standing still!)

Setting standards

Once we have decided on the measure, we need to decide on the required standard, or level of expected performance. Notice how these statements provide the standards (or required levels of performance):

■ If travelling more than 200 miles you should ensure that you have a full tank of fuel before you start (structure).
■ Ensure that your engine revs do not exceed 6500 rpm at any time (process).
■ Ensure that your speed is not less than 40 mph and not more than 70 mph on the motorway (outcome).

It is helpful to apply these now to healthcare settings (after all, not everyone drives), so on an acute ward:

■ There should always be at least one qualified nurse on the ward (structure).
■ Health record entries should be in black ink, signed and dated (process).
■ Patients should not have a length of stay greater than 2 weeks for X condition (outcome).

Note that setting arbitrary standards can be dangerous. For instance, a professional group may feel that 90% compliance with a criterion is an acceptable standard, but that means that they are happy with one in 10 cases not receiving the best available care! If you were one of those 'cases', how would you feel about this standard? So, unless you have good reason (such as research evidence) to back you up, always choose 100% as the standard.

Clinical effectiveness principles

Standards and criteria should conform to the principles of clinical effectiveness. Clinical effectiveness can be thought of as a process of applying the best available knowledge, from research, clinical expertise and service user preferences, to achieve optimum processes and outcomes of care for patients.

From this we see that three elements are required to develop standards and criteria in line with clinical effectiveness.

■ Research evidence.
■ Clinical expertise.
■ Patient preferences.

Research evidence should be used as a sound foundation to healthcare services. There are many sources of research evidence available including those available online (see Chapter 9 for details). You may wish to contact your NHS organisation's library administrator and ask about access to online evidence databases if you are not familiar with these.

The value of clinical expertise should not be discounted when developing standards and criteria. How can you ensure that clinical expertise is incorporated into your standards and criteria? It is important to gain consensus among all the professionals in your service area that the standards and criteria you have selected are acceptable. This is important as results of your audit project may not be accepted by your colleagues if they do not agree with the standards/ criteria that you adopt.

Finally, service users preferences are the final aspect that should not be ignored when developing standards/criteria. Their perspective can be very different from your professional perspective. Where patient preferences are not at odds with clinical preferences, why not include both in your audit? If there is an area where patients and professionals do not agree, then a facilitated discussion could be used to agree consensus. Remember that service users are experts in their care.

SMART principle for criteria

Whatever method you choose, criteria should always be:

- Specific.
- Measurable.
- Achievable.
- Relevant.
- Time related.

Measuring performance

Once your audit project group has agreed on your criteria, now comes the time to look at measuring how your practice compares with the criteria.

Understand the process that generates the data

Usually the data you collect for audit will be generated by a structure/process/ outcome. It is important to understand how the data is generated, since you will be making changes to the structure/process/outcome. When changes to a service are made without a full understanding of the structure/process/outcome, there is a real danger of making things worse! For instance returning to the car metaphor, if your vehicle had trouble getting up to 70 mph on the motorway, simply putting more fuel in the tank would not solve the problem. You would likely need to get the engine serviced or repaired.

Keep things simple – collect the minimum necessary data

Resist the temptation to collect extra elements of data 'because it would be interesting to see'. The data you collect should be enough to say with accuracy to what extent the care measured complies with the standard set. If you are embarking on audit without much experience, you could talk to your local clinical audit department to get examples of good and bad data collection forms. This should help you.

There are some major legal and national reasons for only collecting the minimum data. The Data Protection Act (1998) specifies that, amongst other things, data must not be used for purposes other than for which it was originally obtained. Since quality improvement and service review are included in the functions of NHS organisations, the use of patient data for clinical audit is allowed. However, the Caldicott recommendations (1998), state that NHS staff requesting information should justify the purpose for its collection, and use the minimum patient identifiable data. For example if you were auditing waiting times for a service, collecting information on each patient's age, sex, and ethnic origin would be a waste of time, and probably violate confidentiality and Caldicott principles. You may wish to talk to your organisation's Caldicott Guardian to find out the local arrangements and guidelines for confidentiality of data.

Designing tools for data collection

Once you have decided on what data to collect, you need to plan how to collect it. Often, you will design a paper (or electronic) tool to collect the data. Data collection forms need to be very carefully designed, as the right data is crucial! The data you collect must be precise and essential, the best fit for your purpose. It may include either/both of these forms:

■ Quantitative data (numbers) – this is required to answer how compliant care is with standards.
■ Qualitative data (text) – this can help to determine why a case was compliant (or not) with standards.

Ideally, you should distil your data collection to a series of questions, which you can answer for each case. The responses to these questions should be yes/no or an explicit measurement, for example:

■ Did the patient receive attention within 2 hours of arriving at the department? (quantitative – number).
■ What did the patient find most/least satisfying about the service they received? (qualitative – text).
■ What degree of flexion did the patient achieve in the knee? (quantitative – measurement).

Piloting the data collection tool

Always pilot the data collection tool. This is perhaps the single largest pitfall that audit project teams might fall into when collecting data. No matter how long you spent over your data collection tool there is always the risk of omitting an element that you didn't think of. Piloting the tool saves heartache later on – do you really want to look through all your cases again to pick up one element of data you missed?

Piloting a data collection tool is really quite easy and needs attention to these areas, simply:

■ Get your project group together, with all the people who will be involved in the data collection (where possible).

- Spend half a day looking through a handful of cases and make any changes to a master data collection tool.
- Document the changes in your audit report – this shows to others that you are being systematic.

To help you in this task ask your audit department to help you pilot the data collection tool.

Sampling

The most reliable form of audit is to collect data from every case of care. In situations where data is collected electronically, little effort is usually required to extract the data from the computer system. Establishing a good relationship with your organisation's information department is invaluable in these cases.

Where data has to be collected manually, it is often not feasible to collect details for every case. Manual data collection is extremely time consuming. Statistical sampling techniques are useful to provide a result that can be accepted subject to confidence limits. However, when deciding to select a sample, much thought should be given to what sample is best taken as each could yield different results, for example summer/winter samples, end of year/month samples, time of day samples. Randomisation to collect a sample can be helpful but remember that continuous data sets are most useful to establish the natural variation of a process of care. Again you could ask your audit department for help on determining the correct sample size, if you think you need to use sampling.

Converting data into knowledge

You need to decide how to analyse and interpret the data before you start collecting it. Visualise what you want to see in your audit report. What kind of graphs or tables do you think would be suitable for your need? Check with your local audit facilitator or statistician for different ways of presenting data.

Statistics

For the majority of clinical audit work, not much more than percentages is required to establish the degree of compliance with the standard. Some knowledge of confidence levels is useful, especially when sampling data. Knowledge of statistical process control theory is also useful to understand variations in the data. Remember to keep it simple. If you do not feel confident about the statistics you will collect, consult your local statistician or audit facilitator who may be able to help you.

Reporting and presenting your findings

Most clinical audit projects will result in some sort of report or presentation. You are most likely to be called on to 'present' after the data has been analysed but before improvements have been agreed upon.

Remember that your audit report will likely be read by others who have no idea what you have been up to, so make sure that you put the detail in. Assume your audience knows nothing and then you will fully explain everything that needs to be there.

If called to present at a meeting, always rehearse your presentation. Remember even the most experienced public speakers rehearse their presentations beforehand. If presenting, try to think in terms of ideas, rather than writing a manuscript and reading it word for word. Most people think in terms of ideas in normal everyday conversation and you will sound more natural this way.

Resist the temptation to design the presentation before the report is written as you still need a written report. If you do not complete the report first your potential risk for sending an incomplete message at the presentation is much higher.

MAKING IMPROVEMENTS

Making improvements is the hardest part of the clinical audit cycle. While the NHS has always been subject to change and improvement, the difficulty of changing the way that you, a colleague, or a team works should not be underestimated (see Chapter 3). Simply feeding back the results of your audit will not result in significant improvement. Although feedback is beneficial, used alone it is a weak tool for changing things. You need to distil your audit findings into an action plan.

Findings, conclusions, recommendations, action plans

Once knowledge about the level of performance in relation to your set criteria is obtained, you now have to set about discerning how to improve it. This is really about asking the question 'why?' For instance, if the data showed that 80% of cases are compliant with the criteria, then questions from this could be:

- Why was the compliance not 100%?
- What, if anything, is common to the 20% of cases that were not compliant?
- What can be learned from the 80% of cases that were compliant?
- How can we change our processes/structures to improve our result?

It is unlikely that you will be able to answer these questions yourself. A full understanding of the process of care is required first of all. A worked example indicating how the findings from audit can be forwarded is shown in Table 10.1.

Recognising barriers to change

Just as a sprinter runs differently from a hurdler, you need to adapt your 'running style' according to the barriers you face.

It is generally recognised that organisations face pressures to change and pressures to resist change. These pressures often cancel each other out to form a 'status quo' (see Figure 10.2). Simply increasing the pressure to change results in the pressures to resist change becoming greater 'to compensate' and so the status quo remains. It is more beneficial to analyse and reduce the pressures resisting change, so that the changes can be more readily achieved.

Table 10.1	Using findings, conclusions, recommendations, action plans to improve the service after data collection in audit		
Term	**Example**		**What's missing**
Finding	We noted that the quality in this service area was not good		Everything
Conclusion or recommendation	The department/service area should do better to improve quality We need to do better to improve quality		Clear direction
Action	Person X should do this specific action to improve quality		Timescale and resources
Action plan	Person X should take this specific action to improve quality by this deadline, using these identified resources		Nothing(!)

Figure 10.2
Pressures and drivers for change can cancel out one another in an organisation.

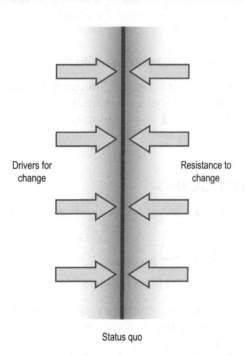

Drivers for change

Resistance to change

Status quo

How can you do this? One way is to list the known factors for 'keeping things the same way' within your audit project group. You can then look at the best way to tackle these or overcome them. You may also need to widen out the discussion and involve other members of your service area in this activity. Your clinical audit department may help to facilitate a discussion around possible barriers to change.

Sustaining improvement

Since we are being systematic in improving things, we need to be systematic in ensuring that things continue to improve. How can we do that?

Re-audit to confirm changes

'Closing the loop' is a phrase commonly bandied about regarding audit; this really means re-auditing an area to confirm changes.

As well as a process to improve the quality of care, clinical audit is very valuable when used to prove that the quality of care has improved. It is important, therefore, that you re-audit the area to confirm that things are indeed better, and therefore 'close the loop'.

When should you re-audit?

Re-audit is of most value once the changes proposed in your action plan have been implemented. Consider the pace of change. What if the changes have not been implemented? Then the re-audit will likely bring up the same conclusions, recommendations and actions that you toiled over to produce the first time round. Why re-invent the wheel?

How should you re-audit?

Generally, it is best to compare like with like, so using a similar sample and the same audit tool and analysis method is recommended. Remember to use the re-audit cycle also to improve the quality of care – it is entirely appropriate to make further recommendations and actions as a result of re-audit data.

KEEPING AUDIT GOING

Clinical audit is a cyclical process, so needs to be kept going.

Developing enthusiasm for audit

Arguably, the main ways to develop enthusiasm for clinical audit are to ensure that:

- Each and every audit project results in sustained quality improvement.
- Quality improvement as a result of audit is 'shouted out' to all relevant staff.
- All staff feel that they can contribute to the clinical audit programme.

Sustaining quality improvement

Having a continuing series of regular audit meetings is key to sustaining an audit programme. At these meetings, spend time looking at the quality of the audit projects your service area has put together. There are various tools available to help you do this; see Appendix VI in 'Principles for best practice in clinical audit' (NICE 2002) for a checklist to evaluate the quality of clinical audit projects and programmes. Also, make sure you monitor the progress of action plans that have arisen from your audit projects as making change is just as much part of the cycle as writing reports.

Dissemination ('shouting out') of learning from audit

Completed audit projects, especially those that have resulted in improvement, can act as a powerful motivator for other healthcare professionals. If your audit project has resulted in a significant quality improvement, then blow your own trumpet! Make use of the facilities in your organisation for dissemination of information to raise the profile of your project. Maybe the principles that you used to make improvements from your audit can be transposed to other areas in your organisation. Good quality audit projects should also be considered for publication in professional journals and displayed/presented at conferences, taking into account data protection and confidentiality issues of course.

Engaging all staff in clinical audit programmes

Your NHS organisation should make training in clinical audit skills available to staff. Tap into this training to increase the skills and knowledge of yourself and your colleagues.

The main way to engage staff systematically is to move from a 'voluntary' approach to participation, to a culture where audit is embedded into everyday practice. Motivation for audit will not be sustained if the 'usual suspects' are continually roped in to audit after audit!

Remember that audit is always easier the second time around, so engage staff that may have been involved before if you are auditing for the first time. In turn you will be able to help your beginner auditing colleagues when you gain some experience yourself.

Reflective questions:

- Do you know what your organisation's clinical governance arrangements are? If you wanted to engage in audit activity how might you access them?
- What would be the advantages of using patients/service users in an audit project in your particular practice area? Do you know how to link up with the Patient Advice and Liaison Service (PALS) co-ordinator or support worker in your area to action patient and public involvement in your audit project?
- Can you identify a suitable area in your practice that might benefit from audit? What might an audit in this area achieve? What information might you seek? How might you action the audit? What support might you draw upon?

REFERENCES

Caldicott recommendations 1998
Online. Available:
http://www.dh.gov.uk/PolicyAndGuidance/InformationTechnology/
PatientConfidentialityAndCaldicottGuardians/Caldicott/ImplementingCaldicottRecommendations/
fs/en?CONTENT_ID=4015633&chk = 6qDZh/
27 April 2004.

Department of Health 1998 *A first class service*. HMSO, London.
Data Protection Act 1998 HMSO, London.
Institute of Medicine 1992
  Online. Available:
  http://omni.ac.uk/browse/mesh/C0025072L0025072.html
  26 April 2004.
Irvine D, Irvine S 1991 *Making sense of audit*. Radcliffe Medical, Oxford.
National Institute of Clinical Excellence (NICE) 2002 *Principles for best practice in clinical audit*. Radcliffe Medical, Oxford.
  Online. Available:
  http://www.nice.org.uk/pdf/BestPracticeClinicalAudit.pdf
  27 April 2004.

RECOMMENDED READING

Health and Social Care (Community Health and Standards) Act 2003 HMSO, London.
* This sets out the role of the Commission for Healthcare Audit and Inspection (CHAI) and the Commission of Social Care Inspection (CSCI).
i-medicine – Clinical audit, effectiveness and governance resources
  http://www.hta.nhsweb.nhs.uk/execsumm/summ601.htm.
* Lots of useful information for would be auditors.
Don't forget guidance produced by your professional organisation.

11 Legal influences on practice

Elizabeth Stallard

LEARNING OUTCOMES

The learning outcomes for this chapter are for you to gain an understanding of:
- ■ The legalised framework of service provision.
- ■ Duty of confidentiality to service users/others.
- ■ Requirement for accurate note-keeping.
- ■ Need for your ethical/professional conduct.
- ■ Whistle-blowing.

INTRODUCTION

As a practitioner of an allied health profession (AHP), you need to have a clear understanding of the law that governs the delivery of your work with service users, and how your practice is influenced as a result.

LEGAL FRAMEWORK

As an AHP it is important to understand the confines of the legalised framework of service provision in which you practise. Your role can be analysed as follows:

- ■ Do I have a duty/responsibility/power?
- ■ What is it?
- ■ To whom do I owe a duty/responsibility?
- ■ Have I fulfilled/exercised it?

Furthermore you may have several roles at once:

- ■ Professional.
- ■ Employee.
- ■ Expert.
- ■ Self-employed.

It is important to note that these roles can exist in tandem, e.g. you are always a professional, but as an employee you have an additional role; you may also give evidence in court as an expert.

Professional

Your role as a professional overrides whatever your employment status. The Health Act 1999 (Section 60) gave a distinct group of healthcare professionals their status as self-regulating professions. These practitioners became known as allied health professionals (AHPs) governed by the Health Professions Council (HPC).

Health Professions Council

Under the Act, the HPC was set up to regulate AHPs in the United Kingdom (UK). It is an independent body which sets and maintains standards of professional training and the performance and conduct of healthcare professions (www.hpc-uk.org). The HPC aims to:

- Safeguard the health and well-being of service users.
- Maintain a register of qualified competent healthcare professionals.

The HPC runs committees dealing with:

- Investigation of complaints/allegations.
- Conduct/competence.
- Health.
- Education/training.

Duties and powers of the HPC

Complaints or allegations about a registered AHP can be referred to the HPC as holder of the register which they will investigate. The HPC concern themselves with matters affecting their aims and if they decide that there is a case to be investigated, there is a structure of relevant committees to deal with this investigation. As an example the education and training committee would consider cases involving a lack of training.

Following investigation the HPC have power over AHPs to impose fines together with their other sanctions of reprimand, imposition of conditions on an individual's practice, suspension and finally de-registration of the practitioner.

The HPC therefore oversee what you do, whatever your role, whether as an independent practitioner or as an employee.

Professional bodies

AHPs are generally members of their own professional bodies which regulate the practice of their particular profession by publishing a Code or Guidance dealing with practice, conduct and behaviour in the UK. Failure to comply with these standards will result in investigation by your own body and/or the HPC. It is important that you know your own body's requirements concerning the standard of professional behaviour expected of you. Each of these documents is updated from time to time to reflect changes in health and social care. As a practitioner you are responsible for adhering to the most recent publication in this respect.

Employee

You have a common law duty to your employer who is responsible for your actions but you also owe a duty to service users and other health or social care professionals. What is the legal position if someone complains about you? Much will depend upon the type of complaint:

- Has harm been caused?
- Is there a breach of ethics/conduct?

Harm

If you directly or indirectly harm someone they can claim compensation for the injury; for example if you supply faulty equipment, or a colleague injures their back when you leave them on their own to move and handle a heavy piece of equipment or a service user. In most cases the claim is against your employer because they are responsible for your actions. The legal expression for this is vicarious liability. If you happen to be employed by the NHS then you are covered by what is known as NHS Indemnity.

If this happens, your name will feature in the resultant case and your version of events will be required but legally and financially your employer is responsible, so your employer will deal with and pay any claim so no contribution will be required from you. In this kind of circumstance, your employer may wish to discuss the matter with you to assess:

■ Why there was a problem.
■ Do you need further advice/training?
■ Are there other undiscovered problems?

In serious cases employers will commence disciplinary proceedings against you or they may refer you to your own professional body and/or the HPC. You are personally responsible for dealing with this and referral to your own professional body is essential. Membership of a union may be useful if personnel issues are involved as the union generally pays for legal fees. However, you can represent yourself or use your own solicitor but you will have to pay your own legal fees and they can be considerable.

Breach of ethics/professional conduct

What then if professional conduct is questioned? Any complaint to your employer and your professional body/HPC will be against you personally and not your employer. Vicarious liability and NHS Indemnity do not apply since it is your professional conduct that is in question and your employer is not responsible for that. It might be said your employer knew about your behaviour and did nothing about it. In that case the complaint will be against both of you but there will be two claims, one against you and one against your employer, so you will still be held responsible as part of this process.

Expert

The Courts regard AHPs as experts and value their help in establishing facts or assessing a person's needs. You can be asked to write a letter/report setting out your views and to attend Court to give your views in person. This is known as giving written/oral evidence. As a result of your involvement by either providing a written report or combining such a report with a Court attendance, you will be entitled to charge a fee for the work that you have done.

First steps

If you are asked to provide a report/give evidence, ask yourself:

■ Is it my area of expertise?
■ Who is making the request?

- What type of report is required?
- Is a visit/examination necessary?
- Does my employer agree to me dealing with this?

Once you have established the basics you can begin to prepare your report and this depends upon the type of report requested.

Compensation claims

People are aware that they can claim compensation for injuries or losses that they have suffered. To win a case they have to prove negligence (see Figure 11.1). As a practitioner either a Claimant or Defendant may request a report from you, or you might be asked to provide a joint report as the request comes from both parties. In this instance you are a joint expert, receiving instructions from both parties and you must communicate in identical terms with both.

The request may be for a report upon professional negligence, e.g. an AHP failed to intervene in treatment/intervened incorrectly and injury has resulted (see examples in Figure 11.2). As a member of the same profession you will be asked whether opinion supports what transpired. If opinion supports events, the claim will fail, however, if opinion does not support events the claim will succeed.

Alternatively in a case where someone is making a claim for the cost of treatment/care/equipment, you may be asked to assess their needs and the costs. A visit and probably an assessment of the situation will be required.

Once legal proceedings are commenced, the Civil Procedure Rules govern how you proceed (The Civil Procedure Rules website – www.dca.gov.uk/civil/procrules_fin/). Rule 35 states that you are a Court expert with an overriding duty

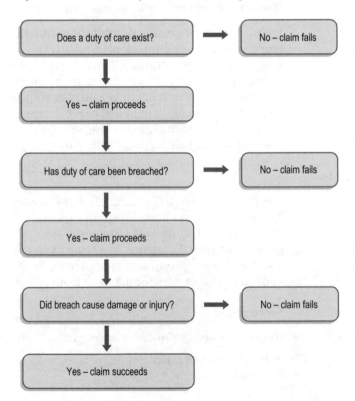

Figure 11.1 Compensation claim flow chart.

to the Court rather than to the person requesting the report. Your report must be as fair as possible setting out not only any issues which support your case but also those which do not.

Rule 35 also sets out what a report should contain and what your duties are. Courses are available to professionals who wish to become proficient in this area of practice and there are also registers of experts that you can join on application. For details consult The Register of Expert Witnesses: www.the-expert-witness.co.uk; the Expert Witness Institute: www.ewi.org.uk; The Society of Expert Witnesses: www.sew.org.uk.

Insurance/occupational health reports

Requests for this type of report will come from:

- Insurance companies.
- Employers.

In these instances you will be asked to assess a person's needs or to provide a copy of a previous assessment. This could be because an insurance claim is being made under a person's own/someone else's policy or the person is finding it difficult to carry out their job. How does confidentiality apply? If you have treated the service user previous to when the request for the report comes in, they have to consent to disclosure. If you have not seen the service user before,

Figure 11.2
Examples of professional negligence claims resulting from breaches of duty.

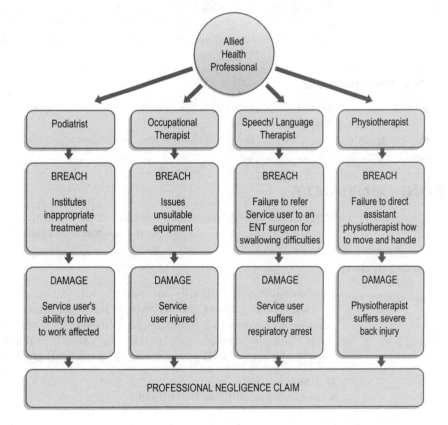

technically there will be a breach of confidentiality in giving the insurance company/employer information. In this instance however the individual can be taken to have consented by arriving for the appointment.

If you have already carried out an assessment and an insurance company/employer asks for a copy, under the Access to Medical Reports Act (1988), you must ensure the service user agrees to this and that they have been told:

■ What is happening.
■ That they do not have to agree.
■ That they have the right to alter the report/correct errors before disclosure.

Self-employed

Your duty here is to the individual/body seeking your services but as an AHP, your duty is also to the individual service user. The benefit of being an independent professional is that you can choose your work but the disadvantage is that you are solely responsible for your professional practice and any complaints or allegations will have to be dealt with by you alone.

Obviously as a self-employed AHP, you are still governed by your own professional body and the HPC but any complaint against you will feel more personal. In serious cases it may affect the amount of work referred to you.

Summary

Although your working roles may vary, you always owe a duty to those around you and must be careful to exercise it at all times. Any complacency may result in complaints to your employer, your professional body and ultimately the HPC, all of whom regulate your practice and can influence it profoundly.

Reflective questions:

■ *What risk management issues should be addressed when drafting a protocol which permits students to work for the first time in the community?*
■ *A colleague slips on coffee you spilt in the corridor. Who does that person sue?*

CONFIDENTIALITY

Service users expect you to keep information confidential. The duty arises in various ways; it is important to know the sources and extent of your duty.

Sources of duty

Confidentiality is primarily an ethical duty rather than a statutory duty although many statutes and regulations do insist upon confidentiality in specific cases. The duty to a service user applies whether you are employed or work for a voluntary agency such as advising carers for the Alzheimer's Disease Society or a local MIND group. Duties of confidentiality are imposed by:

■ Statutes.
■ Regulations/statutory instruments.

- Legal precedents, i.e. past legal cases.
- HPC.
- Professional bodies.
- Contracts of employment.
- Contracts for services.
- Ethical duties.

There is a common law duty (law that has been made by judges over the years), to maintain confidentiality. You must not disclose information and you must store service users' records securely; this would mean for example that leaving records in the boot of your car which is stolen, would be a serious breach of confidentiality.

The HPC and your own professional body provide guidance on confidentiality; however as an employee, your employment contract will contain a clause dealing with this. If you are self-employed then a common law duty of confidentiality applies unless it is included in any written contract for your services.

Exceptions

In going about your duties as an AHP there are going to be occasions when you will need to disclose confidential information to other people. You could not possibly carry out your job if you were not able to discuss a service user's care with other health or social care professionals/colleagues. There are other circumstances in which disclosure of confidential information is necessary and these are discussed below. If you do consider that there is a need to disclose, you need to carry out your own three-stage test:

- Have you the right to disclose information?
- Can you justify your decision to disclose?
- Can you disclose only necessary information?

Even if someone asks for information you do not have to comply and not all of the information you may possess will be relevant to the request so you have to be selective. An example would be if you were asked if someone is fit to work and you know their driving ban has been lifted, revealing the existence of the ban is irrelevant and would breach confidentiality.

If you are unsure about disclosing information then you should discuss it with your manager/the HPC/your professional body or you could obtain your own legal advice.

Can I disclose information?

Yes, if the following criteria apply, as discussed below:

- Service user agrees.
- Service user's best interests served/necessary for their care.
- Statutory duty.
- Court order.
- Public interest.

Service user agrees

If a service user agrees under the Data Protection Act (1998) you can disclose information but you must ensure that they understand:

- What you are going to disclose.
- Who you are going to disclose it to.
- What the information is going to be used for.
- Any possible consequences.

How do you know if a service user is capable of agreeing; for example, they may be psychologically incapacitated, confused or under 16 years of age? To help, there are criteria for determining capacity for agreement. To meet these criteria, you need to be satisfied that the service user can:

- Receive/retain the information.
- Believe the information.
- Weigh the information, balancing the pros/cons.

Case precedent: Re C (Adult: Refusal of Treatment) 1994 WLR 290 (McHale et al. 1997).

If you are in doubt about a service user's capacity to give consent, you must seek a second opinion, e.g. from a consultant psychiatrist – where there is a mental health problem, their assessment will dictate how you proceed dependent upon that service user's capacity. Whatever the outcome of your discussions or assessments you must record them in the notes. If particularly personal information is to be disclosed, the service user's signature in the notes would be desirable by providing proof that the consent has been given.

Mental health problems

A service user with a mental illness needs to meet the criteria above. Service users with serious mental health problems may still be capable of consent to the disclosure of information. If the person refuses, the only occasions where you can proceed are when the disclosure is necessary for example in order to save life or serious harm, to ensure improvement in their condition or prevent deterioration in physical or mental health. They may have a representative, legal guardian or carer who you can consult and who may be able to consent on their behalf, for example if the service user has a profound dementia.

Children

The criteria for disclosure also apply to children. The case precedent for this is Gillick v West Norfolk and Wisbech Area Health Authority 1985 3AER 402 (McHale et al 1997), where a mother (Mrs Gillick) took exception to doctors giving contraceptive advice to girls under 16 years of age. The Court decided that doctors could give confidential advice to under-16s provided the child had sufficient understanding to enable them to comprehend fully what was proposed. If a child is already protected by the Court and the child can consent, it would be wise to involve the Court. A child's age must not be the deciding factor since one child of 17 may be incapable of consenting due to lack of experience/education but another of 14 years may be capable of consenting.

Best interests/necessary for healthcare

Inability to discuss a case with other care professionals would render your job impossible since others need to know confidential information about a service user to give treatment/care. If a service user objects to a disclosure that is vital for their healthcare you can disclose the information but you should forewarn them. An example of best interests would be when a child reveals abuse to you in a paediatric setting but asks that you keep this a secret.

Statute

The Human Rights Act (1998) gives a right of privacy to individuals (Article 8). In cases involving public bodies, e.g. education authorities/primary care trusts/prisons, a claim solely under the Act can be brought by an individual but the claim will be against your employer. An individual can claim under the Act against you personally if they are making another claim against you, e.g. for a personal injury.

The Court has power to prevent disclosures and if this has already occurred to award compensation. This compensation will be paid by your employer if the claim is made against them but if it is against you then your indemnity insurance will pay it and this may have an effect upon the level of premium that you pay each year.

Certain Acts and Regulations require confidentiality to be maintained (e.g. Data Protection Act 1998) whilst others order that there must always be disclosure (e.g. Police and Criminal Evidence Act 1984, Misuse of Drugs Act 1971). Generally a service user has the right to have disclosed to them information held about themselves. Disclosure can be withheld if it would cause serious harm to the service user or someone else, if it contains personal information about someone else or if it would prejudice law enforcement or national security. Disclosure could be refused if someone with a mental illness wanted to see their notes but seeing them could seriously aggravate their condition.

You should be familiar with the various legal provisions and act accordingly. You should always clarify with someone appropriate if you have any doubts before disclosing information or withholding it.

Court orders

Courts can order witnesses to attend hearings to give oral evidence or produce documents and you must comply with this. An order of this kind is called a Witness Summons under Civil Procedure Rule 34, or a subpoena, and failure to attend will result in a fine/imprisonment (McHale et al. 1997). If a Court makes such an order you should obtain a copy of this and read it carefully. Make sure you check for:

- Any time limit stated.
- Any documents/information that are required.
- What else is required of you.
- Whether you can comply at all or in the time stated.
- Date/time of any hearing.

If you cannot comply with an order or you think it is unclear you should contact the Court for clarification without delay and it may be wise to take legal advice through your employer, professional body or union.

You or your employer may disagree with the Court that disclosure is justified; if so you can refuse under the Data Protection Act (1998) and the Data Protection (Subject Access Modification) (Health) Order (2000) but you will have to give evidence to explain why. Such evidence could be that serious harm to the physical/mental well-being of the service user would be caused. It will arise in sensitive cases and you may only wish to discuss the reasons for your refusal with the Judge. Legal advice is strongly recommended in such cases.

Public interest

Revealing information can be justified if there is a real/serious risk of injury or harm to either the service user or any other person. There are restrictions on this disclosure (Case precedent: W v Egdell 1990 1AER 835; in McHale et al 1997). W had been convicted of manslaughter, violence/multiple killings and was detained in a secure hospital under the Mental Health Act (1983). His solicitors asked Dr Egdell, a Consultant Psychiatrist to prepare a report for the Mental Health Tribunal. The report concluded he was highly dangerous and his solicitors dropped his application to the Tribunal. However Dr Egdell thought that the report should be sent to the Medical Director of the hospital and to the Home Office. W applied for an injunction to stop him doing this. The Court said that the report should be disclosed since there was a real and serious risk to the public. The Court considered that the following restrictions should apply to such necessary disclosures and they should happen only:

- Where there is a real/serious risk to the public.
- For as long as the risk lasts.
- If disclosure is to a person with a legitimate interest in receiving the information.
- To necessary information.

As an AHP for example, you might experience a service user disclosing suicidal intent or intention to harm someone else. You need to action this, but remember if you reveal irrelevant information you would be in breach of your duty of confidentiality.

Breaches of confidentiality

If you do breach confidentiality and this was considered unjustified, action may be taken against you depending upon the seriousness and adverse consequences of the breach. Such actions include:

- Employer disciplinary proceedings.
- Termination of contract of employment.
- Referral to your professional body.
- Referral to HPC.
- Legal proceedings for compensation.
- Criminal proceedings if breach prohibited by statute.

The duty of confidentiality should never be overlooked or taken for granted. Before you breach confidentiality you should firstly make sure that you possess all the relevant facts (not assumptions) and that your decision to breach confidentiality is underpinned by any relevant law. Others may pressurise you to change your mind but that pressure should be ignored and only if further information comes to light need you review your decision.

Summary

Confidentiality is a major issue for all AHPs with many complex dimensions. Always be sure of what is expected of you with regards to confidentiality and if in doubt seek advice from someone more expert than yourself before you jeopardise this important concept.

Reflective questions:

■ A service user tells you in strictest confidence that he is a class A drugs user. What should you do?
■ How can the duty of confidentiality be balanced against the public interest?

NOTE KEEPING

Professional notes are essential for a service user's care, the purpose being to document information about their health (Data Protection Act 1998).

Compiling notes/form filling can be tedious but analysis of clinical/non-clinical errors shows that communication through record keeping is a major cause of errors (London National Audit Office 2001).

The types of data that can be considered as notes and an indication of what they should contain are shown in Figure 11.3.

Why is note keeping so important?

Notes should provide a new team member with the detail necessary to enable provision of continuity of care. Your absence on holiday or sick leave should not prevent other AHP practitioners from working with the service user.

Figure 11.3
Professional notes – data types content.

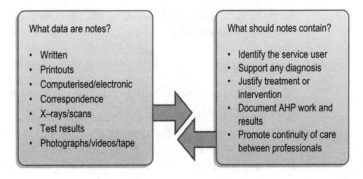

What data are notes?

• Written
• Printouts
• Computerised/electronic
• Correspondence
• X–rays/scans
• Test results
• Photographs/videos/tape

What should notes contain?

• Identify the service user
• Support any diagnosis
• Justify treatment or intervention
• Document AHP work and results
• Promote continuity of care between professionals

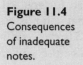

Figure 11.4
Consequences
of inadequate
notes.

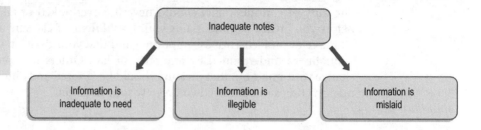

Example 11.1

A service user needs a grab handle to use the toilet safely but you as the visiting occupational therapist forget to record the priority rating. The provision for the service user is overlooked and they injure themselves. You are liable for this injury.

Inadequate notes will compromise a service user's care. This could happen in three ways, as shown in Figure 11.4.

Inability to access information from notes will prevent the delivery, promptness and continuity of care to the service user. Furthermore any shortcomings in the notes you read will affect your professional practice. This could lead yourself or your colleagues to notice your or someone else's inadequacy in their notes and disregard them (if they are there at all), leaving them to form their own judgements. This affects the delivery and continuity of care to the service user, duplicates effort/confidence and standing of specific service professionals will be undermined (see Example 11.1).

Inaccurate or inadequate notes may also result in disciplinary proceedings by your employer, professional body and/or the HPC. In serious cases this can result in civil or criminal proceedings.

The aim of notes

Your notes should aim to:

- Assist in quality of care, treatment and support of a service user.
- Communicate with other professionals.
- Provide clarity about treatment/advice/plans/outcomes.

Compiling notes (see Figure 11.5)

Both the HPC and your professional body have requirements in respect of record keeping (www.hpc-uk.org).

Self-analysis

After making an entry in notes it is wise to review it against these criteria:

- Does it meet any required standards/principles?
- Does it contain all that it should?
- Is recourse to your memory necessary in the future as the note is incomplete?
- Would you mind if the service user or a Judge reads it?

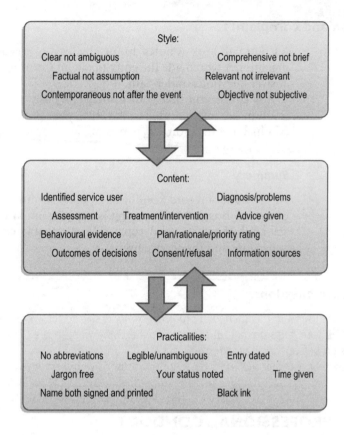

Figure 11.5 Considerations when compiling notes.

Style:
Clear not ambiguous   Comprehensive not brief
    Factual not assumption   Relevant not irrelevant
Contemporaneous not after the event   Objective not subjective

Content:
Identified service user   Diagnosis/problems
    Assessment   Treatment/intervention   Advice given
Behavioural evidence   Plan/rationale/priority rating
    Outcomes of decisions   Consent/refusal   Information sources

Practicalities:
No abbreviations   Legible/unambiguous   Entry dated
    Jargon free   Your status noted   Time given
Name both signed and printed   Black ink

Problem areas

Altering notes – by you

This should never be done. Alteration of notes may be a disciplinary matter and in serious cases can be a criminal offence, e.g. attempting to pervert the course of justice. Remember also that deleted/amended computer records can always be retrieved.

Do not insert information retrospectively as if it were written at the time. You must still note the missing information however by inserting it instead at the next available space together with a note explaining why the entry is not in the correct place. You should date (and time) your entry with the date/time you are actually making it. This clarifies what has happened.

If you record incorrect information you can put a line through it (do not obliterate it though) and sign alongside this line, noting the correct information at the next available place.

Altering notes – by the service user

Service users/others on their behalf can ask to see notes and have copies of them under the Data Protection Act (1998) and Access to Health Records Act (1990). They may disagree with a factual entry and have the right to ask for it to be amended or deleted under Section 14 of the Data Protection Act (1998). If you agree you can amend the entry as explained above; however if you disagree you cannot amend the entry but must insert a separate note that the service user disagrees with the entry.

Litigation and complaints

A Court will look at notes during any legal proceedings and they will need the practitioner who made the entry to attend Court in person to give evidence and answer questions under oath.

Any suggestion that your evidence is false or that your record is false can result in it being reported to the HPC, your professional body or the police for criminal investigation, e.g. perverting/attempting to pervert the course of justice.

Summary

Never think of record keeping as a purely administrative task or just a question of ticking boxes. Note keeping is a professional duty that reflects both your standard of practice and your ability to enable continuity of work with your colleagues and the service user.

Reflective questions:

- *A service user with mental health problems commits suicide. You were the last person to see them alive but your notes are not up to date and the police want to see them. Should you make your notes up before handing them over?*
- *Review your notes for the last 5 days. Are you satisfied with them if you were called to Court?*

ETHICS/PROFESSIONAL CONDUCT

Ethical and professional considerations underpin your role and these will be more difficult if the service user is vulnerable or unable to express their wishes. Ethical issues always arise and must be shared since you will be in a vulnerable position if you act alone (see Example 11.2). Your decision must be informed as illustrated in Figure 11.6.

Figure 11.6
Ways to inform decision making on ethical issues.

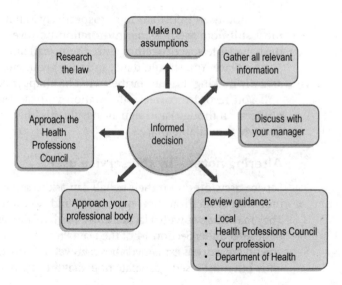

Example 11.2

A service user is dying but their family does not want them to know. They ask you if they are dying. Confidentiality is an ethical issue here. It is often left to the professional to decide but if other professionals are involved you must liaise with them first.

Allocation of resources

Training requires you to assess need but realistically it is hard to meet everyone's needs at the same time. The law/any regulations may not help. They may for example assume a higher level of resources than exists in your area, or they may presume applicable criteria which then render your professional decisions worthless because resources/criteria can vary from locality to locality and from time to time. Courts will not dictate how resources should be allocated and consider that the greater good should prevail. A case that influenced this was R v Cambridge Health Authority, ex parte B (a minor) 1995 23 BMLR 1 CA (McHale et al 1997). B was a 10-year-old girl with non-Hodgkin's lymphoma and then acute myeloid leukaemia who had undergone two courses of chemotherapy, total body irradiation and a bone-marrow transplant. She relapsed and the doctors thought that no further treatment could be usefully given apart from palliative care and that she had 6–8 weeks to live. The father obtained a second opinion that was more favourable to B's survival. The Health Authority refused to fund this further treatment and the father asked the Court for their decision. The Court said that it was not entitled to investigate the merits of the Health Authority's decision or to judge how a limited budget should be allocated to the maximum advantage of the maximum number of patients. An example of how this might apply to an AHP is shown in Example 11.3.

Example 11.3

Mr X demands a hydrotherapy pool to help him but there is no money available. To provide it, 100 other service users would have no physiotherapy. A Court is likely to say that he cannot have the pool, as others will suffer unnecessarily.

Service users who are promised particular help/equipment will become frustrated if there is no real prospect of receiving it. If they are employing you, they will be unhappy if you fail to consider their budget. The potential of your expertise in these instances is devalued in providing a cheaper option that is fit for the purpose.

Implementing decisions

When allocating resources, record the issues, decisions, rationale and whether the service user agrees. In tricky cases or where there is a lack of consent it might be best, if you are a junior AHP, to seek the advice of a more senior practitioner to show a consensus of professional opinion.

A Court might be asked to overturn your decision if someone disagrees with it and the Court will examine your documentation to review the issues. This underlines the need for comprehensive records which cause you no embarrassment.

Professional conduct

It is important to realise that service users will not always co-operate with you or appreciate your help. In some instances a service user may try to hurt you or themselves, for example an older person in an acutely confused state. You should pre-empt any difficulties by preparing for the unexpected.

Your behaviour is crucial since if you upset others this will affect your relationship with the service user, their family and other professionals. Familiarise yourself with the guidance issued by the HPC/your own professional body.

Training

You have personal responsibility to undergo training/continuing professional education to fulfil your role which can change over time. You should undergo training to deal with any situation that arises including violent or difficult situations in order to protect both service users and yourself (see Example 11.4). Information, guidance/course details can be obtained from the HPC, your professional body, the NHS Executive (www.doh.gov.uk) and if you are in employment from your employer as well. As an employee without necessary training, you can approach your employer who should provide it. The law requires employers to protect the health and safety of their employees and others who might be affected by the way they go about their work under the Health and Safety at Work Act (1974). If they do not, then the employee could resign and claim unfair/constructive dismissal.

Example 11.4

As an occupational therapist you work in a rehabilitation setting with older adults and enabling food preparation is part of your role, but you have no training in food handling/hygiene. A service user subsequently contracts food poisoning. You are vulnerable because you held yourself out as an expert when you had no training.

Risk assessment/record keeping

You should be aware of any local policies dealing with incidents, their management and documentation. Clinical governance within the NHS provides for clear lines of oral/written communication, particularly in difficult situations (www.doh.gov.uk/clinicalgovernance/). Failure to pass on relevant information will be traced to you and will affect your professional relationships. If you identify risk and fail to note it you may be held personally responsible for any resulting harm. The service user's records provide evidence of the steps taken to assess risk, any plan to eradicate/minimise it and how you propose dealing with it. You will be more vulnerable working in the community, particularly when visiting service users in their own homes.

A useful risk assessment should be:

- Comprehensive.
- Documented.
- Detailed.
- Objective.
- Acted upon.
- Disseminated.
- Kept under review.

Incidents

Violent situations can necessitate control of the situation or occasionally restraint of the individual. In acting in the best interests of the service user and protecting yourself, the law says you should not use excessive force.

During or after an incident you may need assistance from colleagues, other professionals or the police. If you are in doubt about the situation you should always seek help. Make sure that you familiarise yourself with local policies dealing with incidents, their management and documentation.

Finally, having dealt with an incident, you will need to:

- Tell your employer.
- Note it officially.
- Note it objectively in the service user's notes.
- Complete additional necessary paperwork (accident report book, incident form).
- Inform those who need to be told.
- Liaise with other professionals.
- Review risk assessments.
- Keep your own diary entry.

Consequences

The effects of misconduct or unethical decisions will vary and depending upon the seriousness a range of outcomes can result (listed in Figure 11.7).

Figure 11.7 Outcomes of misconduct or unethical decisions.

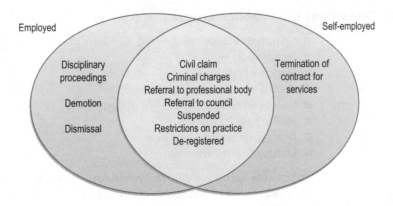

Employed

Self-employed

Disciplinary proceedings

Civil claim
Criminal charges
Referral to professional body
Referral to council
Suspended
Restrictions on practice
De-registered

Termination of contract for services

Demotion

Dismissal

Your professional expertise will be undermined if the ethical implementation of your practice or your conduct is not up to the required standards and the consequences can be severe.

Summary

Ethics/professional conduct are at the heart of professional practice and professionalism. As an AHP you need to be clear of the standards of behaviour expected of you and how to deal with the ethical dilemmas that you may face.

Reflective questions:

- *Review a previous violent situation. What could have been done to prevent it?*
- *You visit a housebound service user. You look at the notes and see that during past visits the family have been violent. Do you continue with your visit?*

WHISTLE-BLOWING

In exposing or disclosing malpractice some people have been sacked, demoted or victimised. They are called whistle-blowers since the process usually involves breaching confidentiality in some form. Example 11.5 describes a case of whistle-blowing.

Example 11.5

A new nurse at a care home was worried about the quality of care. She talked to the Managing Director's personal assistant and was told to put it in writing. Nine days later the nurse told the (then) Social Services Directorate who visited the home. The concerns were valid. The nurse was dismissed and made a claim to the Tribunal who said the disclosures (internal and external) were both protected and reasonable; she received £23 000 compensation.

The Public Interest Disclosure Act (1998) (see Figure 11.8) now provides protection to those who make such a disclosure. They should not be sacked/victimised and will receive compensation if they are. The Act does not cover self-employed workers or volunteers.

What areas does malpractice cover?

- Criminal offence.
- Negligence.
- Breach of contract.
- Breach of administrative law.
- Failure to comply with legal obligation.
- Miscarriage of justice.
- Danger to health and safety.
- Danger to the environment.

The quality agenda of clinical governance means that raising concerns with team members or your manager is important, the purpose being to identify risks and

Figure 11.8
Aims of the
Public Interest
Disclosure Act
(1998).

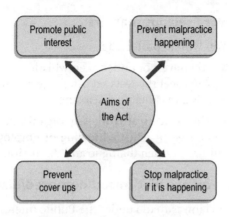

Table 11.1	Types of disclosure; where they may be addressed; criteria for use		
Type of disclosure	**To whom?**	**Criteria?**	
Internal	Line manager/employer. If another organisation is involved disclosure should be made to them	Must be in good faith and have reasonable suspicion that malpractice has happened, is continuing or is likely to happen	
Ministerial	If employed by the NHS/ public body you can disclose to the Government Minister responsible	Must be in good faith and have reasonable suspicion that malpractice has happened, is continuing or is likely to happen	
Regulatory	Applies to bodies regulating particular matters such as Local Authorities, Health and Safety Executive, Inland Revenue, Social Services Inspectorate, Financial Services Authority. Known as 'prescribed regulators'	Must be in good faith and you believe the information/ allegations are true	
Wider	Police, TV/radio, internet, newspapers/journals, etc. MPs, Assembly Members (Wales), Scottish Assembly Members	Not done for personal gain Comply with any of the following: • Reasonably believed you would be victimised if issue raised internally or with the prescribed regulator • Reasonably believed a cover-up was likely and there was no prescribed regulator • You had raised the issue internally or with the prescribed regulator	

manage them although there may be an explanation for what you perceive as malpractice.

Should you make a disclosure?

Assess the situation carefully: much will depend upon the seriousness of the malpractice and your relationship with those responsible for it. To receive protection you have to comply with certain criteria in the Act; these are shown in Table 11.1.

Very serious matters

You will be protected if:

- You have not undertaken whistle-blowing for personal gain.
- You meet the tests set out for regulatory disclosures.
- It is a reasonable disclosure.

Public Concern at Work is an organisation that offers advice to people who wish to engage in whistle-blowing or employers who need advice in developing a culture of open dialogue and discussion (www.pcaw.co.uk).

What happens if you are victimised/demoted/dismissed?

A claim is made under the Public Interest Disclosure Act (1998) by application to the Employment Tribunal (under Section 3). It will decide whether disclosure was justified and award compensation which usually represents your financial losses. If you are dismissed you can also apply for an order allowing you to keep your job (under Section 8).

In the case of wider disclosures the Employment Tribunal will look at:

- Who was disclosure made to?
- How serious was the concern?
- Does the risk/danger still exist?
- Did disclosure breach a duty of confidence the employer owed a third party?
- Was the response of the employer/prescribed regulator reasonable?
- If disclosure was raised with the employer was any whistle-blowing policy used or should it have been used?

Help and guidance are available for those concerned about malpractice or in cases where disclosure has been made and victimisation has resulted.

Summary

Whistle-blowing in the public sector has been brought to the attention of the media, being reported sometimes favourably and also less so in recent times. If you feel you are in a position where whistle-blowing is indicated to protect the public or workers, ensure you are clear of your legal position.

Reflective questions:

- *You help in a voluntary run organisation working with children, but no police checks have been carried out on any of the volunteers. What should you do?*
- *What is your organisation's whistle-blowing policy? Where can you access it?*

CONCLUSION

This chapter has examined some key areas of legal concern that have immediate and important implications on your practice as an AHP. Ensure you are clear about where the legal boundaries to your practice lie and where you might seek help if you have any queries.

Useful websites

Health Professions Council
www.hpc-uk.org

Campaign for Freedom of Information
www.cfoi.org.uk/whistle.html

Public Concern at Work
www.pcaw.co.uk

Department of Health
www.doh.gov.uk

Clinical Governance
www.doh.gov.uk/clinicalgovernance

The Society of Expert Witnesses
www.sew.org.uk

The Expert Witness Institute
www.ewi.org.uk

The Register of Expert Witnesses
www.the-expert-witness.co.uk

The Civil Procedure Rules
www.dca.gov.uk/civil/procrules_fin/

REFERENCES

Access to Health Records Act 1990 Stationery Office, London.
Access to Medical Reports Act 1988 Stationery Office, London.
Data Protection Act 1998 Stationery Office, London.
Data Protection (Subject Access Modification) (Health) Order 2000 Stationery Office, London.
Health Act 1999 Stationery Office, London.
Health and Safety at Work Act 1974 Stationery Office, London.
Human Rights Act 1998 Stationery Office, London.
London National Audit Office 2001 *National Audit Office: Handling clinical negligence claims in England HC403 Session 2000–2001*. London National Audit Office: 3 May 2001.
McHale J, Fox M, Murphy J 1997 *Healthcare law text and materials*. Sweet and Maxwell, London.
Mental Health Act 1983 Stationery Office, London.
Misuse of Drugs Act 1971 Stationery Office, London.
Police and Criminal Evidence Act 1984 Stationery Office, London.
Public Interest Disclosure Act 1998 Stationery Office, London.

RECOMMENDED READING

Department of Health 1996 *NHS indemnity – arrangements for negligence claims in the NHS*. Catalogue No. 96 HR0024, Department of Health, London.
Finch J 1993 *Speller's Law relating to hospitals*. London, Hodder Arnold.
Foster C, Peacock N 2000 *Clinical confidentiality*. Monitor Press, Suffolk.
Health Professions Council 2003 *Standards of conduct, performance and ethics*. 034/HPC/A5.
Jordans 2003 *Civil court service*. Jordans Publishing Limited, Bristol.
Montgomery J 2002 *Health care law*. Oxford University Press, Oxford.
NHS Executive 1998 *Safer working in the community: a guide for NHS managers and staff on reducing the risks from violence and aggression*. Royal College of Nursing, London.
Stauch M, Wheat K 1998 *Sourcebook on medical law*. Cavendish Publishing Limited, London.

PART 3 Professional influences on practice

Conclusion

Lyn Westcott and Teena J. Clouston

The third part of the book has examined some influential forces that shape contemporary practice for AHPs.

The quality agenda (Chapter 8), tracked back to the Bristol inquiry as this marked a critical incident in undermining public trust in the health sector. The chapter discussed how, as a result of this case, the practice of all health workers has changed incorporating a duty to demonstrate quality. This was explored further from the professional level, in terms of self-regulation for health and social care. Implications of the quality agenda for the individual AHP were outlined.

In 'How to be an evidenced-based practitioner' (Chapter 9) you may have noticed how some familiar research concepts from education have been applied

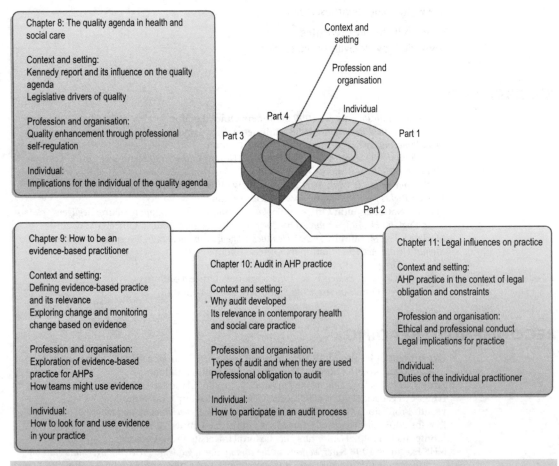

Chapter 8: The quality agenda in health and social care

Context and setting:
Kennedy report and its influence on the quality agenda
Legislative drivers of quality

Profession and organisation:
Quality enhancement through professional self-regulation

Individual:
Implications for the individual of the quality agenda

Context and setting

Profession and organisation

Individual

Part 4

Part 3

Part 1

Part 2

Chapter 9: How to be an evidence-based practitioner

Context and setting:
Defining evidence-based practice and its relevance
Exploring change and monitoring change based on evidence

Profession and organisation:
Exploration of evidence-based practice for AHPs
How teams might use evidence

Individual:
How to look for and use evidence in your practice

Chapter 10: Audit in AHP practice

Context and setting:
· Why audit developed
Its relevance in contemporary health and social care practice

Profession and organisation:
Types of audit and when they are used
Professional obligation to audit

Individual:
How to participate in an audit process

Chapter 11: Legal influences on practice

Context and setting:
AHP practice in the context of legal obligation and constraints

Profession and organisation:
Ethical and professional conduct
Legal implications for practice

Individual:
Duties of the individual practitioner

Part 3 Summary Professional influences on practice

within the professional practice domain. You can now think through what evidence you have seen applied to practice and how you may advance this process. Most importantly you will have read why this is so vital for AHPs.

Audit in AHP practice focused on a particular quality mechanism that is widely utilised in health and social care. The potential of this to reflect best practice has been explored together with an overview of different types of audit tools. The chapter has highlighted how AHPs are obliged to engage in audit and the advantages that this can bring.

Legal influences on practice may have discussed some concepts that were less familiar or more fragmented in your knowledge base in terms of your work as an AHP. The chapter brings together important legal influences and constraints on a range of day-to-day practice issues. The text set out to help you understand the wider statutory elements together with professional and ethical dimensions.

The figure on page 182 provides a brief summary of key issues considered throughout Part 3, highlighting their relevant to the individual practitioner, the professions and organisations in which they work, together with the context and settings of practice.

PART 4 First steps into practice

Introduction

Lyn Westcott and Teena J. Clouston

This fourth part of the book is designed to examine some key areas that will help you understand and reflect on how to best think through a suitable career path for your own personal and professional need, and gives an overview of some key skills needed to secure an AHP post. Chapter titles are:

- Preparing and developing your work as an allied health professional (Chapter 12).
- Securing the right post (Chapter 13).

As with the previous parts of the book, to help you organise and make sense of your thinking and understanding of these important issues, we recommend that you consider the issues from three perspectives. Although it is natural to think at an individual level, the fullest dimensions of career development can only be recognised if consideration is also given to a professional/organisational perspective and the wider context of health and social care provision.

In order to make sense of Part 4, you are advised to bear in mind the three perspectives outlined above. This will help you understand why the text is relevant to your individual situation and career choices. These themes are revisited within the conclusion and summary found at the end of Part 4, which includes an illustration of key areas within each chapter under these headings.

12 Preparing and developing your work as an allied health professional

Ritchard Ledgerd

LEARNING OUTCOMES

■ Promote reflective, practice-based pre-registration student experiences.
■ Investigate the various employment options available to newly qualified allied health professionals.
■ Identify the important features of a first post that promote self-development and professional growth.
■ Explore formal, informal and post-registration learning and development opportunities that facilitate professional autonomy and identity.
■ Explore the factors influencing long-term career progression.

INTRODUCTION

Starting work as an allied health professional (AHP) is a thrilling prospect; you will be filled with excitement, trepidation and apprehension. There has never been a better time to step into the ever-changing world of health and social care. Your path is littered with opportunities and endless possibilities all designed to provide you with a varied and fulfilling career as a healthcare professional. You will have to make a variety of personal and clinical decisions that will be based on the sound reasoning skills you have acquired during your education. This chapter will explore the various options that you may wish to consider before embarking on your journey as a new graduate allied health professional with its subsequent impact on your post-qualifying career options.

REFLECT ON YOUR ACHIEVEMENTS

Some people consider that a person's career as an allied health professional (AHP) starts after they have completed their degree or when they commence their first clinical post. To some extent this is true; however it could be argued that the process actually started a long time before the professional qualification was awarded. A person's career as a potential student and subsequently a health professional student cannot be overlooked. For many years people have been working incredibly hard to qualify as an AHP. The months spent considering what career to choose, investigating what the work involves, attaining the pre-entry qualifications and starting the degree course takes many years of planning and hard work. Reality bites when people embark on their career as a student – the actual complexity of the subjects to be studied, the lengthy fieldwork/ practice placements (not always near home), deadlines, examination preparation, juggling finances and paid work, attempting to retain a social and family life – to name but a few. It is important to congratulate yourself on all the achieve-ments and experiences you have had as student; whether positive or negative they have been useful in shaping your practice as a qualified AHP in the future.

It is also important to acknowledge the valuable friendships and networks you have established during your time at university. Many of the people you have met during your course will form lifelong friends and also professional colleagues in the future. It goes without saying that although the allied profes-sions are expanding in numbers, it remains a relatively small 'professional world' and you can expect to meet people again when you least expect to!

As you say goodbye to your career as pre-registration student, it is important to reflect on the experiences you have had and where your current aspirations lie. It can be a cathartic process and will enable you to gain a clearer idea about your future aspirations as a qualified practitioner.

PREPARING FOR YOUR VOYAGE

Planning your career as a newly qualified professional is not an easy process; like all historical explorers there are lessons to be learned from mapping certain routes and paths. View your expedition as a voyage around the globe. It is a big place spanning many opportunities, currents and directions. As you navigate through your journey you can at least be reassured that you have made some preparatory plans that will enable the crossing to be as smooth as possible. This chapter does not seek to define or prescribe any career maps, but aims to assist your packing and planning before you set sail. Furthermore, this chapter aims to provide you with a compass to ensure that you develop the skills of a seasoned traveller with the ability to plan ahead and prepare for a variety of professional journeys.

Packing and re-packing for the journey ahead

Some people find it difficult deciding where and how they want to work because they are unclear of their own expectations and aspirations as a qualified practitioner. The majority of healthcare professionals will be familiar with the process of continuing professional development and undertaking a self-review can be a useful starting point in assisting your career decisions – a good technique for future practice as an AHP.

Start by reflecting on your experiences as a student and how they have enabled you to reach this point in your career. Consider how your understanding of the profession has matured over the years, from the time you attended your first lecture to becoming a competent practitioner. You have absorbed a lot of information over the years that have contributed to your knowledge base as a future professional. Reflecting on the theoretical content of the course can sometimes prompt feelings of insecurity about not being able to recall every detail from a particular subject area; this is a natural process and not a time to start doubting your ability to practice. In turn it can offer useful insight into your own learning needs and priorities for the future.

Your practice placement experiences have played a part in shaping your career. Re-reading placement reports will demonstrate how your learning has developed and remind you of the clinical experiences that you have encoun-tered. This review will enable you to identify your own strengths, weaknesses and preferences. It will provide a useful platform for considering what avenues of practice you want to pursue in the future. For those who have compiled and maintained portfolios/reflective diaries of their learning experiences, this should be a relatively simple process and should highlight the usefulness of continuing this practice post-graduation.

Reviewing where you have been, where you are now and what you want to achieve in the future is a crucial component to applying for any job as an AHP. It can also provide a useful aid for interview preparation!

Which vessel to sail in?

Planning where you will work is an important decision. For many years students will have read the large number of advertisements for job vacancies in the journals and the therapy press. Most will have read them with an air of fantasy, dreaming of the post-qualifying life and the options available to them as a registered practitioner with the Health Professions Council (HPC). Suddenly the reasons for reading these advertisements become more legitimate and somewhat urgent. Researching which post to apply for and subsequently accept is a significant factor in your postgraduate development.

There is a 'tidal wave of fear' that seems to grip every student in their final year. Some people will get splashed, others will get completely drenched. The wave of fear is usually invoked by a fellow student passing an interview for their first job midway through the final year. This then generates a level of panic within the whole group who are convinced that there will be no vacant posts left at the end of their academic year. Suddenly people are devoting more time to completing applications forms and updating CVs than actually completing the pre-requisites of their degree programme. This is further exacerbated when one person gets a job that another person wanted, resulting in hostile arguments and the meltdown of previously good friendships.

Do not get marooned by this tidal wave of fear; just because one ship has set sail doesn't mean that there are no more ships available or yet to be built. Keep a sense of perspective during this time, remain calm and consider your options carefully.

When you start applying for jobs is entirely your decision. Some employers start the recruitment processes as early as March and April, for jobs commencing in September. For others, it's an ongoing cycle that lasts throughout the year. Some people will have clear ideas about where they want to work and in which speciality, but the majority are often undecided. The art of applying for jobs is covered in Chapter 13 of this book; however some reference to this process should be made here when considering the impact that your first job has on your future career development.

It is reasonable to suggest that you are making one of the biggest decisions of your career and you should therefore ensure that you have researched all the information you need before applying for a job.

WHAT TO LOOK FOR IN A FIRST POST

You want your first job to offer you a stable platform from which to launch your career. There are basic job components that that you should investigate about your future employer prior to making any application for a job. This list is not an exhaustive one, but should provide you with some areas to consider other than *location* and *salary*.

Starting a job that provides a sound *induction* and *orientation* programme enables an individual to gain an understanding of the environment they will be working in. An induction process can provide a scaffold of support to facilitate your future growth as a healthcare professional. Becoming familiar with local policies, procedures and line management structures within your organisation is important; equally knowing where the toilets and canteen are located is just as crucial. An induction process helps optimise all the learning and support mechanisms available to you as a newly qualified practitioner and may include the opportunity to spend time with other professional colleagues.

If you have spent time undertaking a self-review, you will be familiar with your own learning needs at the start of your career. Ensuring these are developed in a structured manner is vital to your professional growth. Looking for a job that offers *regular support and feedback* will pay dividends in the future. Clinical governance is linked to professional practice and most employers will have *annual appraisal systems* in place to assist your future development as an allied health professional. In addition, it is worth investigating what other support mechanisms are in place; whether it is *formal or informal supervision, peer group review or employment training opportunities*. Most employers will be conversant with the practice of continuing professional development (CPD) and you may want to ascertain how your future employer supports its staff to engage in this activity.

Whether you are going to work in an organisation with a large staff and client group, or a smaller organisation with a uniprofessional focus, you would be advised to consider the *staffing ratio* and *resources* available to its employees.

Advertisements can sometimes be deceptive and if there is an opportunity to visit the organisation beforehand then you would be advised to do so. Some employers can offer a range of *additional benefits* to its staff to promote a healthy work/life balance; this may include recreational facilities, crèche and childcare support, flexible working opportunities and *postgraduate learning resources*, to name but a few. It is worthwhile exploring the selection available to you as a new employee.

Consider what *quality standards* and *clinical effectiveness measures* are used within your employing organisation. Most departments will engage in a variety of measures to enhance clinical effectiveness and good practice. Participating in and designing audits and reviewing service delivery can be both challenging and interesting. You may wish to investigate what systems are in place and how you can contribute as a new practitioner.

Answers to these questions should help you to assess what the job will offer you as an individual and also as a newly qualified practitioner. Whilst these considerations are important, do not forget there is a responsibility for you to demonstrate to your future employer what *you* will offer the post. One of the most important things to remember is that although there is a national shortage of qualified staff, employers still have the *choice* in recruiting the most appropriate person for the job. It is imperative to communicate what you can offer the service, not just what it can offer you.

Where to look?

Professional bodies produce regular publications that usually house a variety of job advertisements. As the world of recruitment continues to expand, it is worth considering alternative ways to search for available jobs.

Some employers choose to advertise vacancies directly to the university courses, so it is worthwhile reading the local advertisement boards within your institution and attending local university careers fairs.

Internet searching is a popular way to locate jobs housed on a variety of independent websites; using a major search engine can help define your search more accurately, for example www.google.co.uk.

Therapy Weekly is a popular publication for some of the therapy professions (www.therapy.co.uk) and also provides some professions with a guide to starting work.

The 'Society' supplement in the *Guardian* newspaper; www.jobsunlimited.co.uk is useful for health and social care vacancies and www.communitycare.co.uk also lists a wide variety of social care jobs.

Recruitment agencies are also able to find permanent jobs throughout the UK and there should be no charge made to you for this service. A useful website is www.agencycentral.co.uk.

Many public sector organisations are going through a period of change and reconfiguration. This can sometimes make finding the name of a particular organisation difficult. The Institute of Healthcare Management (IHM) (www.ihm.org.uk) produces an annual yearbook that lists all health and social services establishments and their respective specialities. This is available for purchase but can also be found in your local library. Alternatively search the NHS website www.nhs.uk for details of local NHS organisations or http://www.ukonline.gov.uk for social services/work listings.

If you are interested in working for a particular employer, it is worthwhile contacting the human resource department or therapy manager to ask to be notified of any forthcoming vacancies.

Which destination to choose?

Irrespective of what profession you have chosen to study, you will have a choice in the range of opportunities available to you. Narrowing these down can be problematic; however the self-review process will provide some insight into where your interests may lie. Choosing your final career destination at the start of your journey would not be realistic; climates, currents and personal circumstances change, all of which have an impact on where you find yourself. Having an idea of where the first leg of your journey will end is more practical and usually prompts people into contemplating which 'professional continent' to set sail to.

Rotational post or static post?

Some professions provide an opportunity for new graduates to rotate through a range of jobs at a junior level before deciding on an area to specialise in. Rotations usually last between 4 and 6 months and, dependent on the type of organisation, can offer a variety of clinical specialities. These types of posts are ideal for people who are undecided about their preferred career options. Revisiting a clinical area as a qualified practitioner is different to being a student and you have the opportunity to implement your skills in a different way. These types of posts are sometimes available at a more experienced grade, ideal for those who remain undecided or enjoy the variety of different clinical environments. A different yet comparable option is to consider a non-rotational/static post. People choosing to work in this type of post can develop their skills in a particular field of practice without having to move around into different clinical environments. It provides an opportunity to build long-term relationships with professional colleagues and dependent on the specialism, longer-term relationships with their clients. There is no recommended option when considering rotational or static posts; both have their advantages. It is a personal decision that should be based on your learning objectives and more importantly your personal preferences.

Career break

Having spent many years completing a degree course some people consider taking an extended holiday before entering clinical practice, others are keen to start work as soon as possible. If you choose to travel the world, start a family or simply take a period of time off, it would be advisable to remain up to date with developments within your professional community. Employers do not usually perceive taking a break at the start of your career as detrimental to your employability. Some professional bodies enable their members to join in an overseas, associate or non-practising category. This ensures you receive all necessary professional updates wherever your location and the various profession-specific websites enable you to access the information at the click of a button. If for any reason your break is longer than expected and you do not feel confident enough to start or return to the clinical field, then contact your local university who will provide further information about government funded return to practice courses.

Further study

Some people choose to continue their education on a part-time, full-time or distance-learning basis immediately after obtaining their first professional qualification; others prefer to spend time 'recovering' from the initial process! It is worth investigating the pre-entry requirements of your second degree before making any definite decisions. A searchable database of postgraduate courses can be found on the internet at http://www.postgrad.hobsons.com.

Private and independent practice

Considering whether to pursue a career as an independent or private practitioner should take serious thought. The majority of professional groups who represent practitioners working in this manner strongly recommend that new graduates gain a high level of post-qualifying experience before contemplating this option. Becoming a confident and expert practitioner may take several years to achieve and is usually the basis for entering independent practice. Your professional body will be able to provide you with further information when you feel that you have attained the right amount of experience to develop your career in this direction.

Temporary or permanent employment?

Many new graduates are tempted to consider locum or temporary employment as a way of solving their high levels of student debt. Whilst locum posts tend to pay more money, the job often requires the skills of an experienced practitioner who is also able to work independently. In addition, reputable agencies do not usually employ junior staff without any postgraduate clinical experience. In 2003, the NHS in England and Wales launched a framework agreement for the supply of temporary AHPs to NHS bodies. This was developed in response to the high level of expenditure made by NHS organisations on temporary staffing. The agreement sought to improve the quality of service offered by the large number of agencies supplying staff to the NHS, in addition to regulating the pay and charge rates made by these suppliers. Provision was also made for the appraisal and development of locum staff, which does make reference to new graduates choosing to pursue this employment option. Further information can be obtained from www.pasa.doh.gov.uk. It is recommended that you consolidate your own professional skills before considering this option and look for posts that will support your own learning and development needs.

Working overseas

Pursuing your career in another country can be a rewarding and life enriching experience. There are endless opportunities available to AHPs in both developed and developing countries. The majority of professional bodies are members of international communities, which support and develop the practice of their respective professions across the world. Some professions also have European representation that focus on the professional identity within the European Union. Whilst working abroad can be a unique professional and personal experience, serious consideration should be made before the process of careful preparation for this experience can begin. Communication is of vital importance and making sure you have a speaking knowledge of the language of the country you choose to work in is crucial. You should also be in good physical and emotional health to work overseas, as your system may be exposed to changes in climate, nutrition, working hours and human attitudes. Your professional skills and knowledge will be challenged every day so gaining some postgraduate experience in the UK would be strongly advised. Research the country you are going to be working in, consider politics, cultural patterns, education systems, financial implications, professional entry requirements, existing support networks and visa restrictions.

Some commercial and charitable organisations can assist with the transfer of UK educated staff to a variety of international communities. The Voluntary Services Organisation (VSO) can provide information about working in a voluntary capacity in a range of developing countries; contact: Enquiries, 317 Putney Bridge Road, Putney, London, SW15 2PN UK (http://www.vso.org.uk). Many of the UK recruitment companies have international offices that frequently place trained staff in permanent and temporary positions abroad.

Gaining some postgraduate clinical experience will ensure you have the necessary skills to practise safely and confidently in another country.

PASSPORT TO PRACTICE

The Health Professions Council (HPC) is an independent, UK wide regulatory body responsible for setting and maintaining standards of professional training, performance and conduct of the 12 healthcare professions that it regulates. These professions are arts therapists, chiropodists/podiatrists, clinical scientists, dieticians, medical laboratory scientific officers (MLSOs), occupational therapists, orthoptists, prosthetists and orthotists, paramedics, physiotherapists, radiographers and speech and language therapists (www.hpc-uk.org).

If you want to work as an AHP in the UK, you must be registered with the HPC (www.hpc-uk.org). When you complete your education you need to ensure that all the necessary documentation and fees have been submitted to the HPC for approval. Under no circumstance can you practise as an AHP without certification from the regulatory body. As the majority of new graduates qualify in the summer months, the registration process at this time can sometimes take a little longer to complete. Many employers make provision for these inevitable delays by employing people to work in a support worker role until their registration is complete. If you perform any work in a support worker capacity, you must ensure you have a job description that accurately describes the work you are undertaking.

Relevant documents and further information can be obtained from the HPC at The Health Professions Council, Park House, 184 Kennington Park Road, London SE11 4BU. Tel: 020 7582 0866; UK Registrations lo-call number: 0845 3004 472; Fax: 020 7820 9684 (http://www.hpc-uk.org).

Tickets, money, passport

Once you have evaluated all the multi-faceted options available to you as you a new graduate entering into professional practice, you will have been able to make some informed decisions about how your career will develop. Having reviewed your recent experiences, identified your current learning needs, explored the possible employment options, considered the available career paths and met the statutory registration requirements you will be able to start your journey as an AHP.

As you embark on your journey, you may want to pack some life essentials to ensure your expedition goes as smoothly as possible:

Pride in your profession

Many people become increasingly forlorn at the prospect of describing what they do for a living. They consider the general public to be misguided about what their professional qualification actually means. This concept seems to haunt many AHPs, which in turn generates a negative, self-fulfilling prophecy. The majority of people will have heard of what you do, but the likelihood of them describing what you do in finite detail is remote. Does a person who works as an engineer actually build engines all day? Does that mean that a civil engineer is a person who is always polite when building their engine? How many jobs have you actually heard about without actually knowing what they involve? The relevant stakeholders know what you do for a living – increased government funding and the expansion of allied health profession services are evident throughout the UK. People need to celebrate what they do for a living, communicate their achievements on a bigger and louder scale and adopt a greater sense of pride in their professional career. Believe in the principle that as long as you know what you do, why you do it and the recipient of your intervention is informed and confident of your professional expertise, then this is all that should matter.

Membership of a professional organisation

Remaining actively involved with your professional organisation enables you to develop a sense of identity within your particular professional community. It can provide support, advice, membership benefits and representation at a national and local level. Some organisations also have clinical interest forums that you can join to help develop your professional practice. Never underestimate how valuable your professional communities are to you as a new graduate.

Practice placements

You may be asked to make room on part of your journey for people who are interested in sharing your expertise and career choices. As the majority of students will remember, the availability of appropriate practice placements was limited due to the shortage of qualified professionals willing to supervise their practice. Remaining involved in student education is vital to the development of your profession and your contribution will be invaluable. As a new graduate you may not feel that you have sufficient knowledge or confidence to supervise someone on a full-time basis; however you can still participate in the clinical education of student on a more informal level. Your local university will be able to provide further information about how to get involved in student education.

Having selected and planned your route as a newly qualified healthcare professional, you can set sail to your first destination. The crossing may not always be smooth; however if you spent time making the appropriate preparations and considered what support mechanisms should be available to you at times of need, then your journey will be a lot safer and more rewarding when you reach your first destination.

Planning your career expedition

Having prepared yourself for the immediate journey ahead, there will become a time when you will contemplate making another journey to a new destination. As you acquire the skills, language and working knowledge of your profession, your ability and confidence to undertake your first post will increase. It is reasonable to suggest that you can only be considered a newly qualified practitioner for a certain length of time after which you will eventually be considered experienced in the practice of your profession. This, coupled with your thirst to develop your expertise in new and different areas, will promote an organic process of change. Your first post is an opportunity to consolidate your theoretical and practical knowledge, the importance of which should not be overlooked or understated.

Mapping where you want to go will become clearer when you have become acclimatised to the professional and organisational requirements of your first post. Some people's expectations change dramatically when they have had an opportunity to experience a range of clinical experiences – never be deterred by these influences as they can often have a positive impact on future career decisions.

Irrespective of your chosen profession, there are a number of fundamental principles to address when considering how, when and where you evolve your career as an experienced health professional. The majority of employers will have a structured appraisal system in place, linked to local clinical governance measures. Appraisals can offer a wealth of learning opportunities and insight into your career development and it is important that you maximise on this two way process. Embracing the feedback you receive and the associated outcomes provides a platform for enhancing your skills as an AHP. It also provides an opportunity for you to share your thoughts on the learning environment that you are working in. Consider the process as an ever-evolving travel guide that reflects the current climate and conditions of where and how you work.

It is important to recognise that ambition should not supersede experience and the adage of not running before you can walk is an important consideration. Enthusiasm should not compromise clinical competence and the ability to perform the role of junior and senior practitioner requires experience. Appraisals and continuing professional development will provide ongoing insight into your skills and clinical ability. Remember that accountability and public safety should be at the forefront of any professional intervention and whilst some people consider the kudos of promotion as important, primary thoughts should be with capability.

Remaining up to date with changes in government policy and legislation is crucial to your career planning; they remain an important part of professional practice. Your time limited experience as a pre-registration student will provide an indication of how quickly working patterns and locations can change! A useful way to remain aware of changes is to read the various professional journals for updates on any significant changes.

CONCLUSION

This chapter could not possibly describe every job permutation available to you as a qualified AHP. Needless to say there a range of professionals working in a variety of clinical and non-clinical environments throughout the world; these include expert practitioners, educators, researchers, project workers, civil servants, professional body representatives, even international managers of independent companies! The majority of people who have pursued these career paths have one thing in common – their ability to reflect. Experience, personal aspirations, competence and confidence are the primary drivers in developing career plans. As an AHP, the world remains a very accessible place. The key to reaching your destination is to plan your route carefully, learn from previous experiences and share your findings with other intrepid explorers. Bon voyage!

Reflective questions:

■ Do you feel confident that you have reflected on your experiences as a pre-registration AHP?

■ Would you feel comfortable in being able to list your experiences, strengths and weaknesses in order to start your career as an AHP?

■ Are you familiar with the variety of search engines available that will enable you to find suitable postgraduate employment?

■ Would you actively participate in local professional body activities to support your development as a new practitioner?

■ Have you considered the various employment options available to you as a new graduate?

■ Could you design a career plan based on your pre-registration experiences and current preferences? Would you be willing to adapt this as you progress through your career?

13 Securing the right post

Helen Hortop

LEARNING OUTCOMES

The learning outcomes that will be explored in this chapter are:
- Discussing when and where to start looking for a post.
- Outlining guidance on which vacancies to apply for and which grade.
- Delineating how to make an application, including how to formulate attractive documentation to support your application such as a curriculum vitae (CV), including why CVs may be rejected.
- Consideration of how to prepare well for an interview including what happens before and during the interview process.
- Guidance on what you might expect from an employer to support decision making on accepting or rejecting a post.

INTRODUCTION

Securing the right post can be stressful both for new practitioners and for experienced job seekers. The purpose of this chapter is to try to remove some of that stress by discussing each step in applying for a post and being interviewed.

WHEN TO START LOOKING

There is no right time to start looking for a job, although undergraduates may be under pressure in the last year of their course, particularly the final 6 months, to start earning as soon as they qualify. If this applies to you, then even when under pressure you need to consider whether it is more important to complete your studies first or to go job hunting. Marianne Bos-Clark (2001), a speech and language therapist, recalled the anxiety felt by herself and fellow students when one of their group was the first to be offered a post. It left her feeling worried that the best jobs would be gone by the time she applied for them. Of course the evidence of one person taking a single job means this will not be true, so it is important to resist the temptation to worry at this stage. Remember you may end up making unwise decisions or compromising your studies at an important time.

WHERE TO START LOOKING

Geographically speaking, the question of where to look for jobs is a matter of personal choice. It may depend on where the family home is, or perhaps you had a particularly successful practice placement, in which case you may wish to return to that hospital or company. When it comes to tracking down vacancies, most of them are advertised nationally in professional journals, but employers can also use local publications or the internet. Other useful sources include the

Therapy Weekly Guide, which is published annually and focuses on new graduate posts for occupational therapy, physiotherapy and speech and language therapy. It is sent to every UK educational institution for these professions. It also gives good advice on the issues covered in this chapter, and this advice is useful to all job seekers (see also Chapter 12). Some organisations may advertise junior posts at job fairs or via flyers sent to universities and colleges. In your final student year it is therefore worth consulting the notice boards for job seekers. Finally, when looking for a post, do not underestimate the value of networking and using that network as a potential source of information about vacancies when they arise (Perlmutter Bloch 1993).

DECIDING WHICH VACANCIES TO APPLY FOR

It is important to think carefully about whether the post that you wish to apply for is the right one for you. Finding yourself in the wrong job may cause you so much distress that you begin to doubt your career choice. Perlmutter Bloch (1993) recognises this when she says 'Many people are concerned right now about you and your future. That's because leaders in business, government, and education recognise how important it is for each and every one of us to find the job we want. This is important both for personal satisfaction and the country's economy' (p. 5).

When it comes to deciding which vacancies to apply for as an allied health professional (AHP), you may wish to consider whether your prospective employer offers rotational posts. These provide an opportunity to continue the learning process in a variety of workplace environments. One advantage of this is that you will have a much clearer idea of the path you wish to follow when the time comes to specialise in a particular field.

Another important consideration, especially for new practitioners, is how much support and supervision they can expect to be offered in their new job. One of the benefits of clinical/practice supervision is that it helps therapists to develop their skills, discover their strengths and become aware of their continuing professional development needs (Moir 2002).

In fact, you should be concerned about a whole range of services offered by your prospective employer. For instance, the College of Occupational Therapists (2002) recommends that the following should be available: 'Induction/ orientation procedures, supervision/support structures, commitment to continual professional development (CPD), in-service training/staff training budget, quality standards and clinical effectiveness measures, staffing/study resources and annual appraisal systems' (pp. 5–6).

The points above include factors that candidates should bear in mind when deciding whether or not to apply for a post. For instance, it is increasingly the case that organisations are acknowledging the benefits of CPD. In connection with this, Investors in People (IIP), the national standard for effective investment in the workforce, was developed in 1990 in conjunction with leading UK businesses. Employers given IIP approval often display a logo on their advertising material to this effect. Taylor and Thackwray (1996) say:

'Subscribing to Investors in People demands the creation of a learning organisation. Most have:

■ A culture that values and rewards learning.
■ Personal and professional development integrated into strategic planning.

- Systems and specialists that are used to enhance personal and professional development.
- Clear development and support offered equally to all staff throughout their time with the organisation and at all stages of their career.
- A clear and well articulated link between development and appraisal.
- Evaluation as an integral part of the personal and professional development iterative loop' (pp. 163–164).

It needs emphasising, however, that searching for a job is like looking for a partner with whom to form a reciprocal relationship: what counts, if the partnership is to be successful, is that each of you meets the requirements of the other.

Although candidates always think of whether they might be selected by an employer, it is interesting to learn that in some cases key decisions are taken by the candidates not employers. Jenkins (1983) discusses one case where . . . 'Of 370 people originally expressing interest, half did not complete an application form. Of the 23 people who were offered posts, over a third did not take up the post' (p. 259). This example illustrates how important it is for prospective employer and employee to marry up their needs by trying to ensure that they each have what the other wants. It is not a simple matter of employers advertising a vacancy and accepting or rejecting applicants. The job seeker also has the power of choice, just like the employer, and this is exercised at all stages from choosing among vacant posts to deciding whether or not to accept the offer of a job.

It should be kept in mind, too, that many professions are classed as being in shortage, particularly within the AHPs. It is clear therefore that the job seeker has the power of choice and can shop around for the best opportunity. Even when a vacancy attracts many applicants, filling it is still a process in which all parties expect their requirements to be met. For the applicants the objective should be not just to get the job but also to find that it meets their needs – in short, that they are happy in their work.

Which grade should you apply for?

It is important to apply for a post at an appropriate grade to your experience. As some posts are difficult to fill, employers may be tempted to attract new staff by appointing them at grades that are too high for their professional profile. This can result in too much responsibility being placed on new recruits. It is important to look for a post with challenges, but they should be ones to which you can rise without undue stress and with the benefit of support and supervision. As a rule, new practitioners should be appointed to junior training grades. This is a national standard set by professional bodies. The Royal College of Speech and Language Therapists Pre-Graduation Pack (2003) states that the purpose of grading is to:

- 'Safeguard individual therapists to ensure that they have the support and supervision they need for their post and that they are not expected to carry out duties or take responsibilities above their level.
- Provide a clear structure to allow for progression and development.
- Safeguard the patient by providing service structures and quality of care to match the level of responsibility' (p. 9).

According to *Therapy Weekly Guide* (2000–2001), 'Therapy posts tend to increase in seniority depending on how much you supervise other people, the specialist nature of the work you do, and the level of managerial responsibility you take on' (p. 20). It is important therefore that prospective candidates consider carefully whether the expectations for any grade of post match their developing skill base, aspirations and competencies.

MAKING YOUR APPLICATION

It is worth pointing out that new practitioners often apply for more than one post at a time and because employers are aware of this practice, there is no need to make a secret of it. It is always better to be honest with your prospective employer. However many jobs you apply for, the application usually has three elements: a letter, an application form (part of which will include a job description and person specification) and a CV. As these documents may be the first contact made with a prospective employer, yours must stand out from the crowd. This is particularly important when there are new practitioners seeking employment at the same time, many of whom will have a similar level of training and experience at this point.

Most organisations have a standard application form. To make sure this is completed as required and that it includes all the information needed, read it closely in order to understand it before you set pen to paper. Making a photocopy to complete as a draft before writing the final version is a good idea. If it says on the form that BLOCK CAPITALS or black ink should be used, either for the whole of it or for particular sections, then make sure that you use them.

A brief and professionally presented accompanying letter on good quality writing paper also helps to give a professional impression. Remember to use the correct ending for your letter. If it begins 'Dear Sir or Madam,' it must end 'Yours faithfully'; if you write to a named person, it should end 'Yours sincerely'. A written or telephoned confirmation that you will be attending for interview also gives a courteous and professional tone to your application.

With regard to CV writing, it is worth noting that the literal translation of 'curriculum vitae' is 'story of your life'. This is an important document which should be continually revised and updated. It should reflect your development as well as being tailored to the post being applied for. The post requirements will be laid out in the job description and person specification that the employer will have sent you, so should be easily at hand. Torrington, Hall and Taylor (2002) refer to a person specification as 'listing the key attributes required to undertake the risk' (p. 172). They also note: 'In addition to, or sometimes instead of, a person specification, many organisations are increasingly developing a competency profile as a means of setting the criteria against which to select. Competencies have been defined as underlying characteristics of a person which result in effective or superior performance; they include personal skills, knowledge, motives, traits, self image and social role' (p. 192–193). When you receive the person specification you will see that it is divided into sections with headings such as 'previous experience', 'qualifications' or 'skills'. There may be sub-sections in which desirable qualities are separated from essential ones. Make sure that you satisfy those conditions that are specified as being essential. With regard to desirable qualities, these are also important, make sure you list the ones you have or anticipate having. For example, if owning and driving a car is noted as desirable and you are currently taking driving lessons then make the employer aware of this. If the person specification says that a degree in psychology is essential and you don't have one, you won't be considered for the post, so there is no point in applying for it. If you think that you do satisfy the conditions, modify your CV in such a way as to highlight your suitability with respect to them.

Different formats of a CV

There are two main formats for a CV, the chronological and the achievement-focused. The chronological gives information about a current or most recent post first, listing the others in reverse date order. The advantage of this format is that it helps to emphasise forward development and growth. The second sets outs achievements in accordance with points listed as essential or desirable in the person specification. This format is most effective when candidates are looking for a first or early post in their career, since it allows them to parade their particular strengths.

Writing your CV

Whatever format you choose, there are three essential elements of a successful CV: these are skills, personal qualities and achievements. After completion of an AHP course, new practitioners have a broadly similar level of skill, which is why it is important to stress qualities and achievements. For example, all graduates in health studies have spent time in a clinical/practice speciality area. To describe that period as perhaps '4 weeks in rheumatology in hospital X' means little. To describe your positive experiences or your accomplishments during that time is much more impressive. For example, 'during a 4-week period in the rheumatology department I completed an audit that resulted in a change of practice which improved service outcomes'.

CV writing, as with so much else, is subject to changes in fashion. Gone are the days when CVs were judged by the number of pages they contained. Nowadays, they should be short, concise and contain only details relevant to the post. These should include full contact details. Employers with several candidates for a post are unlikely to pursue someone difficult to contact. It is a very personal document, so write it in the first person: 'I enclose', 'I wrote', 'my achievement'.

After your personal contact details, it's a good idea to set out a personal profile; for example, 'I am an enthusiastic new graduate eager for the opportunity to improve my skills in physiotherapy.' Following this give an account of your:

- Employment history.
- Educational history and qualifications. If you have a degree, then instead of listing General Certificate of Secondary Education (GCSE) subjects and pass marks, just state the number of passes and their dates.
- Professional qualifications in full and include membership, or student membership, of professional associations and special interest groups.
- Work experience, describing it in a way that complements your professional qualification, especially if you are a new practitioner. A part-time job in a Burger Bar could be turned around to include inter-personal relationships,

team working and customer care. In this way, you will be able to show that your catering experience has enabled you to develop the qualities that your prospective employer is looking for.

Remember to make your CV personal, make it interesting, use 'power' words and use the first person: I planned, I represented, I implemented, and I assisted. Ensure all relevant achievements are listed; but be honest and do not take credit for something you didn't do. If your role was assisting implementation rather than implementing, say so. A misleading statement on a CV can come back and haunt you!

Let us return to those three essential elements of a CV: skills, personal attributes and achievements:

- Skills are what you gain through training, such as teamworking skills, assessment skills, technical skills.
- Personal attributes may include adaptability, creativity and willingness.
- Achievements are signposted by such power words as 'I improved', 'I gained', and 'I delivered'.

Lastly, it is usual to give the names of two referees, their contact details sometimes included in the CV; if they aren't, they will be required on your application form. Unless they have given you their general permission, referees must be consulted prior to each application. It is usual to give one professional reference from your current employer or from a senior member of staff within your college; the other may be a personal or character reference, perhaps from a senior colleague or from someone having status in the community. If you are in employment but you have not given your current employer as a professional referee, you may be asked to explain why not. References provide both a factual check and information on your suitability for the post (Torrington, Hall and Taylor 2002).

Keeping in touch with referees is important. Do not expect someone who gave you supervision on a placement 3 years ago to remember you. Supervisors see many students; unless you were an outstanding or particularly awful one they may have forgotten you! It is to your advantage to ring or occasionally visit your potential referees. This advice applies equally to first and post-registration job seekers.

Torrington, Hall and Taylor (2002) state, in relation to references 'the factual check is fairly straightforward as it is no more than a confirmation of facts the candidate has presented. It will normally follow the employment interview and decision to offer a post. . . . The character reference is a very different matter. Here the prospective employer asks for an opinion about the candidate before the interview so that the information gained can be used in the decision-making phases.' (p. 204)

In practice, both references are usually requested at the same time. In most organisations they are read after the interview has taken place and used as part of the selection process.

Under the Data Protection Act (1998) applicants who are successful have the right to see any references written about them, unless the referee has specifically asked not to allow access. The act, which came into force on 1st March 2002, is being supplemented by the Employment Practices Data Protection Act (2002) from the Information Commissioner. The act is in four parts and part one covers recruitment and selection.

Reasons why CVs are rejected

Sometimes CVs are rejected and candidates not called for interview. This can be for a number of reasons, one of which is that there may be hundreds of applicants for a single post. As part of the process of arriving at a shortlist, it is not unknown for someone to choose at random from a pile of CVs and select only from this small group, leaving the others unread.

If there are too many candidates, a poor first impression given by a CV or application form can result in it being rejected out of hand. The CV may be unduly long, use different typefaces, contain mistakes in grammar, spelling or punctuation or be badly presented. It is always worth asking someone else, perhaps a colleague or a tutor, to read the draft CV, just to give a second opinion about the impression it makes and on ways of improving it.

PREPARATION FOR AN INTERVIEW

Visiting prospective employers prior to interview can provide the opportunity to gain information in an informal environment. Many AHPs arrange a pre-interview visit and this course of action is wise even if the department to which you are applying is one where you were placed as a student. If possible, make an appointment to talk to the head of department; but if this cannot be arranged, then you should at least be able to speak to other members of staff. Many departments have information packs available, and these may be obtained before your interview and studied at leisure.

Some departments arrange open days; if they do, make every effort to attend. Any difficulties in finding the site or locating yourself within it can be overcome with this pre-interview visit, which can also be used as a trial run for the logistics of arriving on time. Remember there is nothing worse than rushing breathless and flustered into an interview room.

It is important to note that that during the visit other people will be gaining a first impression of you as well as you of them. From the moment you arrive on site, anyone you meet may have contact with, or influence in, the department. The receptionist you met very briefly while you waited to be shown into the office may be asked for an informal opinion. As well as making a favourable impression during your visit, it is also a good idea to write a letter of thanks afterwards. Anything that you can do in these and other ways to prepare yourself in advance will increase your chances of being successful on the day.

What happens before and during the interview?

Interviews can be thought of as a conversation with a purpose. In an interview the dialogue is controlled, with more meaningful exchanges than expected from an ordinary conversation. Interviews can be viewed as ritualistic in demanding particular behaviours from all participants, with the process itself standing like an initiation ceremony to the new employer (Torrington and Hall, 1987). Jenner (2000) states that during the interview 'Your prospective employer will be using a range of techniques to discover more about you. They will be aiming to find answers to the following questions:

- Will you be able to do the job?
- Will you fit into the department or section where you will work?

- Are you enthusiastic and motivated?
- Will you be flexible and work well in a team?' (p. 204).

Jenner goes on to highlight that '55% of communication depends on body language, 38% to how you speak and only 7% to what you actually say!' This is certainly important to bear in mind.

Argyle (1988), an eminent writer on interpersonal skills, makes some interesting points on how interviewees should behave. Argyle's opinion is that interviewers seem to prefer candidates who are well-presented and quietly dressed, politely attentive and keen, and they are likely to reject candidates who are rude, over-dominant, not interested or who irritate them! Dress and appearance at interview are important components of an initial impression. The College of Occupational Therapists (2002) recommends that the interviewee should wear something smart but comfortable, interviews being the wrong day to experiment with dramatic hairstyles and colours. If the image you want to project is one of professionalism and competence, then choose clothes that reflect such an image. For instance, it can be distracting if a female candidate wears a very short skirt and is constantly tugging at it to try to keep it in place.

Turning to particular details, it is worth repeating that it is important to try to arrive early for interview, since it makes such a bad impression if you arrive late. While awaiting your turn, try to take the opportunity to sit quietly, calm down and practise managing your stress; don't worry about experiencing some nervous apprehension as this is quite normal before and during an interview.

When your turn arrives you should be greeted in a friendly manner outside the interview room and then taken in to be introduced to the panel members. It may be advisable to wait until they offer their hand to you and to shake it briefly and firmly, smiling at them as you do so.

If you find you are nervous and your mouth goes dry (or you anticipate this), do not be afraid to ask for a glass of water. Try not to cross your legs, fold your arms or generally tie yourself into a physical knot – it only increases your stress. Take the time to sit comfortably, keeping your hands open, either in your lap or resting lightly on the arms of the chair. This should be positioned in such a way that you are able to see all the interviewers. If it is not, then politely ask if you can move it. If you breathe out deeply when you are seated, this should help you to relax.

Each interviewer will ask you some questions. Listen to them carefully and pause and think before answering. If you do not understand, ask for clarification or for the question to be repeated. Look at the questioner, but not to the exclusion of the rest of the panel. Remember the importance of body language. When the panel is finished they should ask if you have any questions of your own. At this time you could ask about opportunities for CPD or about supervision or rotational posts. Panels generally do not mind if you have written some questions down prior to interview – this can then help you remember any important points that are easily forgotten if you are anxious. At the end of your interview, always thank the panel for inviting you to attend.

Keep in mind that an experienced interviewer will make every effort to put you at your ease, it is to everyone's advantage that you feel comfortable. If no such effort is made, then it is worth asking yourself whether this is the right employer for you.

Sometimes, as a preliminary to individual interviews, candidates are interviewed in groups. Your letter of invitation should warn you in advance if this is the case. This type of interview may be resorted to when there are very many candidates for a post. Plumbley (1985) regards group interviews as a way of providing insight into candidates' abilities to:

■ Get on with one another.
■ Influence other people.
■ Verbally express themselves.
■ Think both logically and clearly.
■ Use their past experiences to apply themselves to a new problem.

With group interviews there are two points worth emphasising, the first being that it is much easier to speak up early in the discussion. More people will have gained the confidence to voice an opinion as time goes on and it is more difficult to come up with something original to say. Secondly, try not to appear judgemental, resisting temptation to argue vigorously against someone else's view. Acknowledge a difference of opinion and then present your own.

It may be worth considering whether professional development portfolios should be brought to an interview. These are records of achievements and CPD is becoming a pre-requisite for ongoing registration for all HPC staff (see Chapter 6). Whether they should be presented at interview is a difficult question to answer as there is usually more than one candidate being interviewed in a limited time. Realistically, a portfolio cannot be reviewed in depth, although it can look very impressive to the panel if it is well-prepared. Perhaps you could consider taking it to an informal interview, or offer to leave it for the panel to read after a formal interview.

Finally, here is a recapitulation of some of the main points in this chapter, together with some new ones. First of all, value yourself as a person with skills and qualities and remember that your objective as a job seeker is not just to pay the bills but also to be happy in your work. For this reason ask yourself not just whether you are suited to a particular vacant post but also whether it is suited to you.

When applying for a job emphasise your skills, personal qualities and achievements, and do so in a way that is tailored to its particular requirements. Make sure that anything you write is correct with regard to spelling, grammar, punctuation and choice of words. If you feel uneasy about something you have written, check it or find some other way of phrasing it.

Make a practice run to the interview venue so that you know how long it will take to get there. If you are travelling by public transport, check routes, times, etc. Make every effort to arrive in good time but take with you a contact telephone number and ring to apologise if you are delayed.

First impressions are important, so be polite and courteous to everyone when you present yourself for interview. Try to appear confident, make eye contact, shake hands firmly and with a smile. When answering questions do not ramble but keep to the point. Have some questions of your own in case you are invited to ask them. Dress appropriately.

Be prepared. For instance, most organisations have a web page, so use it to obtain as much information as possible. This will enable you to give informed answers and to ask pertinent questions.

Finally, remember that they probably want you as much as you want them.

CONCLUSION

Securing the right post is a vital part of your professional experience and career development. This chapter has introduced you to some of the practical aspects of preparing for and participating in processes of recruitment and selection, enabling you to make informed decisions of what you might best do and when. Although these processes can be rather daunting, remember that as an AHP you have a lot to offer a potential employer. It is useful to remember that they probably want you as much as you want them as this can give you a great confidence boost!

REFERENCES

Argyle M 1988 *The psychology of interpersonal behaviour*, 4th edn. Penguin, Harmondsworth.

Bos-Clark M 2001 On the fast track. *Royal College of Speech and Language Therapy Bulletin* December: 6–7.

College of Occupational Therapists 2002 *Your guide to starting work as an occupational therapist*. College of Occupational Therapists, London.

Data Protection Act 1998. HMSO, London.

Employment Practices Data Protection Act 2002. HMSO, London.

Jenkins JF 1983 Management trainees in retailing. In: Ungerson B (ed.) *Recruitment handbook*, 3rd edn. Gower, Aldershot, p. 259.

Jenner S 2000 *The graduate career handbook – making the right start for a bright future*. Financial Times, Prentice Hall, London.

Moir D 2002 Advancing reflective practice through clinical supervision. *Royal College of Speech and Language Therapists Bulletin* September: 4–5.

Perlmutter Bloch D 1993 *How to get a good job and keep it*. VGM Career Horizons: a division of NTC Publishing Group, Chicago.

Plumbley PR 1985 *Recruitment and selection*, 4th edn. Institute of Personnel Management, London.

Royal College of Speech and Language Therapists 2003 *Speech and language therapy: the first step, pre-graduation pack*. Royal College of Speech and Language Therapists, London.

Taylor P, Thackwray B 1996 *Investors in people explained*, 2nd edn. Kogan Page, London.

Therapy Weekly Guide 2000–2001 *The essential handbook for all qualifying therapists*. Grange Press, Brighton.

Torrington D, Hall L 1987 *Personal management, a new approach*. Prentice-Hall, London.

Torrington D, Hall L, Taylor S 2002 *Human Resource Management*, 5th edn. Prentice Education Ltd, England.

RECOMMENDED READING

Bradley A 2003 Bradley CVs.
   Online. Available:
   http://www.akc.co.uk/cvtips/index.htm

Fear RA, Chiron RJ 2002 *The evaluation interview*, 5th edn. McGraw-Hill, New York.

Job World. *The Resumé Store International*.
   Online. Available:
   http://www.cvtips.com/

Johnstone J 1999 *Passing that interview*, 5th edn. How to Books Ltd, Oxford.

Stewart J 1999 *Employee development practice*. Financial Times, Pitman Publishing, London.

PART 4 First steps into practice

Conclusion

Lyn Westcott and Teena J. Clouston

This fourth part of the book has developed themes to help you understand how best to take charge of your professional career. It has offered a range of suggestions to enhance your control in determining your career path including practical tips that will make you more knowledgeable and confident in this process.

Preparing and developing your work as an allied health professional (Chapter 12) gave you an overview and understanding of the breadth of opportunities in the context of professional development and growth. This is important as it broadens your focus beyond the immediate factors that may influence your job seeking choices and encourages a more strategic long-term approach to career development.

Securing the right post (Chapter 13) offered you some useful, practical advice on skills required for selecting a post and recruitment. This should therefore help you think through how to secure the post that is best for you and fulfil your desired career plan.

The following figure provides a brief summary of key issues considered throughout Part 4, highlighting their relevance to the individual practitioner, the professions and organisations in which they work, together with the context and settings of practice.

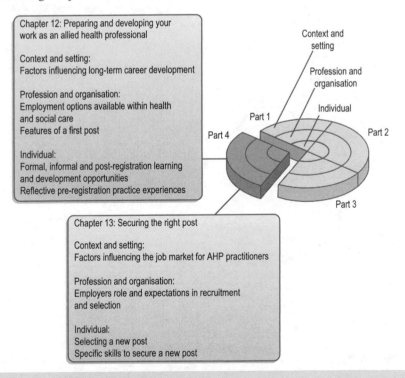

Chapter 12: Preparing and developing your work as an allied health professional

Context and setting:
Factors influencing long-term career development

Profession and organisation:
Employment options available within health and social care
Features of a first post

Individual:
Formal, informal and post-registration learning and development opportunities
Reflective pre-registration practice experiences

Context and setting

Profession and organisation

Individual

Part 1

Part 4

Part 2

Part 3

Chapter 13: Securing the right post

Context and setting:
Factors influencing the job market for AHP practitioners

Profession and organisation:
Employers role and expectations in recruitment and selection

Individual:
Selecting a new post
Specific skills to secure a new post

14 Epilogue

Lyn Westcott and Teena J. Clouston

This final chapter does not aim to introduce new content and ideas as the other chapters have done. It does however aspire to help you think through the important concept of applying the reading of the material to your current and future professional life.

We have brought together writers with important messages and things to say about a number of key themes in contemporary health and social care. We have endeavoured to group these under logical themes, categorised as parts in the text, to aid your understanding of how a complex picture may be assembled and applied to your work. This is because health and social care practice exists in a context of ever-changing, multi-faceted influences and variables. The situation is particularly complicated for the allied health professionals (AHPs) because their foundations are not as deep as those of the traditional perceived workers in this field (i.e. nurses and doctors). The professionalism of the AHP group has been marked by the emergence of the Health Professions Council (HPC), consultant therapists and higher level practitioners.

This book consolidates a new way of thinking for the AHPs, drawing on issues of common interest that we share to shape our quality practice. AHPs are a single group of highly skilled experts drawing on a diverse knowledge base to serve the public in multiplex ways and within a wide variety of settings. We are embracing the innovations of recent years looking for practice opportunities outside the conventional boxes from which our professions emerged. This means we are moving away from the traditional confines of practice seizing opportunities for creativity and innovation in our work.

The recognition of this commonality between the AHP readership led us initially to develop this text as a source that would be equally helpful to any profession, and indeed any individual practitioner within a profession. This is because we all have shared but different needs. This means that readers of this text cannot be inactive; there is a challenge inherent in this book which parallels the challenge of working as an AHP. The reader needs to apply the common concepts introduced here to their own circumstances, profession and practice and use this in turn to develop a unique strategy to continuously update their knowledge base and professionalism. This could include for example developing the knowledge and themes introduced here by supplementary investigation at greater depth, found within more specialised texts in each chapter area.

The book is in line with the contemporary expectation of the AHP as a reflective and autonomous individual, responsible for being proactive in recognising and acting upon their development needs. With this in mind we have drawn the readers' attention to how the information given within the chapters may be applied. This moves the reading on from the individual perspective that we naturally assume when the content of some writing links to our immediate experiences. The summaries at the end of each part of the text therefore highlight the content of each chapter to three domains of interest; with the individual in the centre, their profession and employing organisation surrounding this and finally the wider contexts and settings in which these operate, for example government drivers.

The challenge to our readers is of course an ongoing one; health and social care has changed significantly over our careers and we are sure that it will continue to do so. This is because AHP practice is inevitably symbiotic with government strategy and thinking and both of these are subject to development and change over time. We therefore hope that the concepts within this book will help you forward in your professional journey, wherever you may be now and whatever your destination will be.

Index